For Bruce and Sophie

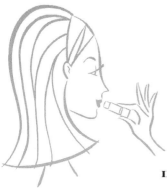

contents

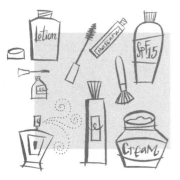
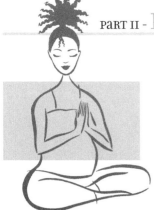

FAST BEAUTY

1,000 QUICK FIXES

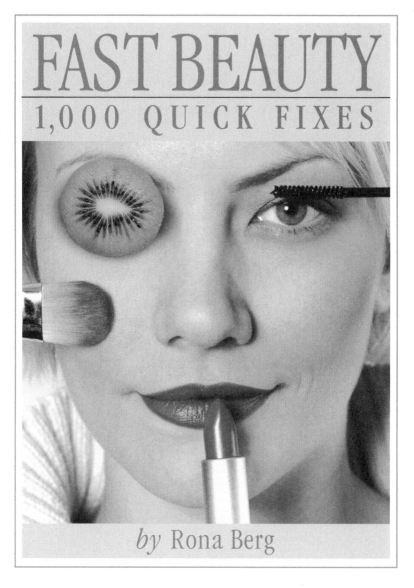

by Rona Berg

WORKMAN PUBLISHING ▪ NEW YORK

Library of Congress Cataloging-in-Publication Data
Berg, Rona
Fast beauty : 1,000 quick fixes / by Rona Berg.
  p. cm.
Includes index.
ISBN-13: 978-0-7611-3472-5
ISBN-10: 0-7611-3472-7
1. Beauty, Personal. 2. Women—Health and hygiene. I. Title.
RA778.B4734 2005
646.7'042—dc22   2005042676

Designed by Janet Parker

Workman books are available at special discounts when purchased in bulk for
premiums and sales promotions as well as for fund-raising or educational use.
Special editions or book excerpts can also be created to specification. For details,
contact the Special Sales Director at the address below.

Workman Publishing Company, Inc.
708 Broadway
New York, NY 10003-9555
www.workman.com

Printed in the U.S.A.

First printing: August 2005

10 9 8 7 6 5 4 3 2 1

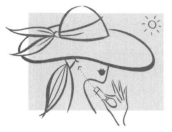
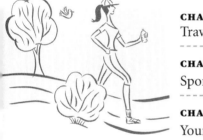
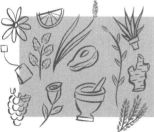

acknowledgments

My deepest thanks to Peter and Carolan Workman, and to my incredible editor, Ruth Sullivan, the best a writer could hope for. Kudos to Paul Hanson and Janet Parker, an amazing design team, and my illustrator, Mary Lynn Blasutta. I'm grateful to Nicki Clendening for her creative publicity ideas, to Kris Dahl and Jud Laghi for being there and for being so good at it, and to Beth Hatem, a research whiz!

I'd also like to thank the beautiful people who helped along the way: Ole Henrikssen, Mark Garrison, Jean and Jane Ford, Bobbi Brown, Sonia Kashuk, Jenefer Palmer, Barbara Close, Linda Nicholas, James Takos, Marie-Laure Fournier, Laura Hittleman, Rebecca James Gadberry, Stacey Miyamoto, Leslie Roth, and Peggy Boulos-Smith. Thanks to the good doctors, Dr. Jeanine Downie, Dr. Diane Berson, and Dr. Carol Livoti for their medical expertise. And thanks to all of the glamorous folks in the beauty industry who have been so generous over the years.

Finally, my deepest gratitude to Bruce and Sophie; my parents, Alan and Sheila Berg; my brothers, Andy and Neil Berg; my sister-in-law, Rita Harvey; and my grandmother, Lillian Berg, who have all taught me so much about true beauty.

INTRODUCTION

Vanity is the true mother of invention. When smooth, hairless legs were all the rage in ancient Babylonia and the Venus razor was still some four thousand years away, women achieved a state of hairlessness by "threading"—positioning a thread between the fingers and teeth, wrapping it around each individual leg hair, and giving it a tug. It worked pretty well if you didn't have much else to do with your time.

Then one day, an enterprising woman who probably had too many goats to tend in the Tigris-Euphrates Valley accidentally spilled some hot wax on her body and, after quickly peeling it off, discovered a quicker way to get rid of unwanted hair. More or less, that's how waxing was born. And to this day, for most women, fast beauty is better.

While looking good is still a top priority, it can be a challenge to fit our beauty needs into our fast-paced lives. In the midst of juggling work, family, social engagements, business travel, and visits to the gym, something's got to give. These days, none of us has time for complicated beauty regimens. But that doesn't mean we don't want great results—fast. It's why I decided to write *Fast Beauty: 1,000 Quick Fixes*, a beauty handbook packed with timeless tips for women who have no time. *Fast Beauty* will cure whatever ails you with a quick and effective Rx that's often right at your fingertips. Whether you don't know what to do, need a quick substitute for what you usually do, or just want to simplify your life, this book will provide fast, easy solutions that work. After all, we live in the land of fast cars and fast food. Why not fast beauty?

The book will pare down your beauty regimen to the basics in the 2-minute face, the 5-minute face, even the 30-second face, when you haven't a minute to spare. It will also help you resolve the beauty fallout that can result from too much stress, work, illness, even medication. It will provide easy solutions to hormonally driven hang-ups that come along with puberty, periods, pregnancy, and menopause. And it will give you the information that you'll need to master all of your beauty meltdowns at the gym, on the road, in every type of weather (frizzy hair, anyone?), and at home with your family. It will even offer some guidance to the men in your lives.

Like a bouillabaisse, *Fast Beauty* is a big soup that's spiced with a dash of folk wisdom, just the right amount of product recommendations, and a few heaping spoonfuls of natural remedies. It will debunk the most common beauty myths, show you how to mop up your beauty messes, tell you how to pinch-hit when you're out of beauty supplies by using ordinary household products, and teach you how to tweak your makeup, hair, and body care to enhance the way you look and feel—in no time! Lackluster hair? Cadaverous complexion? Larger-than-life pores? Cakey concealer? Clumpy mascara? Thinning hair? Razor burn? Cracked heels? Streaky self-tanner? Cold sores? Puffy eyes? Breakouts? Bacne? No problem! Check the index, and you'll find an almost instant solution.

I'll never forget the day one of my elegant colleagues at *ELLE* magazine used the example of her new next-season's sample Yves Saint Laurent coat-dress to teach a life lesson to some of the younger staff. With a rather dramatic gesture (fashion editors are nothing if not flamboyant!), she unbuttoned her dress and folded it back to show us how the collar, hem, and sleeves were secured on the inside with masking tape, Velcro, and safety pins. "Sometimes life leaves you hanging by a thread," she said, "and you just have to figure out a way to hold it together." That's the wisdom this book has to offer. *Fast Beauty* provides inventive ways to patch up those tiny tears in the fabric of life—fast—so that you'll have more time to live it.

In my 20 years of experience in the fashion and beauty industries, I've made it a practice to create and stockpile beauty tips. This book offers the best of the best of these tips. It will show you how to save money, and when it makes sense to spend it. Its approach is meant to inspire you to be as clever and resourceful as my fashion-industry friend. Because when we travel down the road of life, we can always use a good shortcut.

PART I:

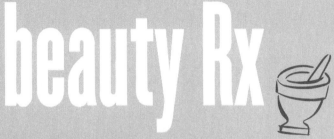

beauty Rx

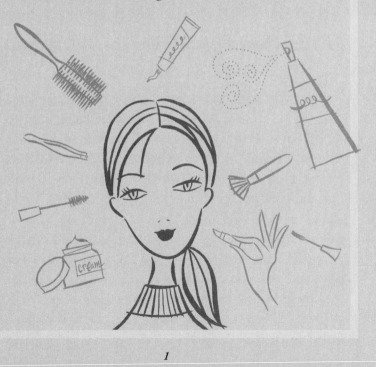

CHAPTER ONE

YOUR BEAUTY CLOSET

Things You Should Never Be Without

VERY BEAUTY EDITOR AT EVERY WOMEN'S MAGAZINE has a beauty closet. For the staff, being privy to its delicious confections is one of the great perks of working there. Whether luxurious walk-ins or just a few shelves, these closets are jam-packed with just about every conceivable beauty product that is sold (or about to be sold) in the United States. It's no wonder the beauty editor's reign as closet queen makes her the envy of the entire staff. For beauty voyeurs—editorial or otherwise—the beauty closet is a fantasy playland. But the coveted closet is a utility at the magazine, too. Well-stocked with items that the beauty editor, editor-in-chief, or publisher may find herself lacking—just before she's

closet beauty

In the magazine's beauty closet, editors can always count on finding the following:

1 A full range of the most up-to-date moisturizers, lotions, serums, and balms

2 Blow-dryers, hair clips, candles, and perfume

3 The current and future season's full makeup palettes—from foundation to lip gloss, and everything in between

4 A tin of balm or Vaseline to add a last-minute lick of shine to cheeks, lips, and décolleté

5 Tools of the trade: makeup brushes, sponges, spoolies, and eyebrow combs

6 A range of dry shampoos, for those moments when washing the hair is out of the question, but a greasy do just won't do

7 Multiple tubes of black mascara, colored mascara, eye pencils, eyeliner, eyelash curlers

8 Lipgloss, for a patent-leather pout

9 Nail files, top-coats, clippers, and polish—in every imaginable color

10 Hair gels, shine serums, waxes, hair spray, creams, mousses and pomades—from Kiehls to Kerastase

11 Hair elastics, ribbons, bows, combs, brushes, diffusers, curling irons

12 Squishy tubes of cheek gel or bronzer, for a rosy flush or a hint of healthy color

13 Eye pillows, essential oils, aromatherapy products

14 Shower gel, loofahs, body brushes, body scrubs

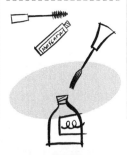

to dash off to a business dinner or black-tie event—the closet is an indispensable prop to looking one's best.

I believe that every woman should have her own version of this beauty closet at home—even if it's just a drawer or two in a back-room dresser. Now, obviously, no woman needs the big candy mountain of a beauty editor's closet, but this chapter will tell you (1) what you'll need for your day-to-day beauty regimen, and (2) the multipurpose items that are basic to every woman's fast-beauty pantry. If you have these items on hand for those momentary beauty meltdowns, it'll save you a lot of aggravation. (Of course, you'll want to supplement these basics with some of the great makeup products recommended throughout the book—these are your closet's secret weapons.) Your beauty pantry will be your updated, more glamorous exemplar of the old Girl Scout motto: Be prepared.

Beauty Basics

Knowledge is power, my Grandpa Sam used to say, and knowing how to care for your skin, choose the right makeup, maintain healthy hair, and put your best face forward can be a really powerful boost to your self-esteem. And once you get the hang of it, it won't take more than five or ten minutes out of your busy day.

When life gets hectic, women who have it together don't suddenly fall apart—and neither will you, if you've got your beauty regime under control, along with a ready stash of basic beauty supplies on hand.

Here's what you need to streamline your daily regimen. Once you've established it, you'll never have to waste another minute thinking about it!

Basic Products For Your Regimen

CLEANSER

Wash your face thoroughly with a gentle cleanser, once or twice a day, depending on your skin type. (If it's oily, twice a day. Once a day will do for dry skin.) *Never* sleep with your makeup on (but you knew that!), and never use soap on your face—no matter what your skin type.

EXFOLIANT

Exfoliation can make the difference between okay and out-of-this-world skin, and it becomes even more important as you get older. Whether you use a glycolic acid cream, a retinoid, or a simple scrub, you're sloughing off the dead skin cells that pile up on the skin's surface, which not only makes your skin feel better, it also enables moisturizer to penetrate better. Perhaps you have more time in the evening to exfoliate, but do it several times a week after washing your face (less frequently if your skin is very dry or sensitive).

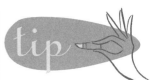

JUICY SKIN

Put a bit of moisturizer in a tiny container (a lip gloss pot or a cosmetics-counter sample jar) and always carry it with you in your purse. Dab a bit on whenever your skin feels dry.

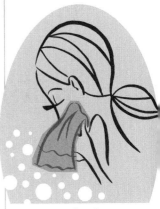

You can slough away dead surface cells with a nubby terry washcloth. Don't rub, just buff lightly.

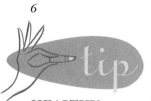

HEALTHY SUNSCREEN

Look for a sunscreen enriched with healthy, skin-saving antioxidants, which are on the brink of proving themselves highly effective sunscreens as well.

MOISTURIZER

Moisturizers contain emollients—occlusive ingredients that seal moisture into your skin—and humectants, which attract moisture. All skin types benefit from a moisturizer, unless you have severe acne. If you need proof, notice how much juicier your skin looks and how much softer it feels after you moisturize. Your skin will benefit most from a product that is compatible with your skin type: Dry skin loves a heavier cream, and oily skin needs an oil-free lotion or gel.

SUNSCREEN

If there's only one piece of advice you take away from this book, it's this: Use sun protection on your face every day, even when the sun doesn't shine. (See pages 130–133.) Choose an SPF 15 sunscreen that contains titanium dioxide, zinc oxide, or Parsol 1789 (avobenzene) listed as an active ingredient. For everyday, choose a moisturizer, foundation, or tinted moisturizer with SPF 15.

EYE CREAM

An eye cream is a worthwhile indulgence. The skin beneath your eyes has no fatty layer, few oil glands, and not much support structure, which is why it wrinkles so easily and needs special care. Pat your eye cream on the undereye area lightly with your fourth finger, which exerts the least amount of pressure. If your skin is oily, look for a gel formulation; otherwise, a silky-smooth, pearly cream is quite nice.

SUPPLIES AND TOOLS

COATED ELASTICS

Have coated, clasp-free elastics on hand to sweep your hair back into a tidy ponytail in two seconds flat. These are preferable to the ones with clasps, because they won't snag or break your hair.

A STASH OF LITTLE CLIPS

Clips will accessorize your look, and smooth down any short stray hairs that refuse to behave themselves, especially on a hot, humid day.

TRIANGULAR MAKEUP SPONGES

A triangular sponge (dampened) not only helps your makeup go on smoothly and evenly, it doubles up for damage control. Use it to soften cakey makeup, smooth flaky spots (around the nose, between the brows), and swab the crease of your eyelid lightly to absorb excess oil before you apply eye shadow. (Pick up a big bag of them—they're really cheap!)

CREAM BLUSH STICK OR TUBE OF CHEEK GEL

By midafternoon, your skin—no matter what color—can look washed out and flat. A little dab of color applied to the apple of your cheek can instantly brighten your face and give you a healthy, natural-looking flush.

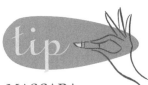

MASCARA SPOOLIE

Makeup artists buy these by the bagful, in drugstores or beauty supply shops. Spoolies are, essentially, little mascara wands used to declump mascara on the lashes and to comb and groom the brows.

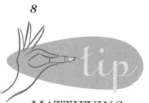

MATTIFYING LOTION

A dab of mattifying lotion is a great way to absorb excess oil and shine, especially on the T-Zone.

EYELASH CURLER

An eyelash curler will open up your eyes like you won't believe. It's easy to use (always curl your lashes *before* you apply mascara, or the lashes can break), and it makes your lashes look more lush even if you don't wear mascara.

BLOTTING PAPERS, OR RICE PAPERS

Blotting papers are perfect for soaking up the oil on the T-Zone around 4 P.M., when oil glands can go crazy. Wonderfully portable, they're great when you're on the go, and they'll leave your skin looking matte and shine-free.

HAND WIPES

Always carry a couple of individually wrapped hand towelettes in your purse. They come in handy for swabbing up mini-messes, removing makeup from your hands, and washing your hands when there's no sink handy. (Choose wipes made with natural ingredients and avoid those with triclosan, which can be drying.)

HARD-PRESSED Q-TIPS

Available in drugstores or beauty supply shops, these Q-tips are great for smudging eyeliner, applying acne medication, and swabbing up makeup smudges on your face. Because the cotton is hard-packed, it won't shed little fuzzy bits on your face that can get in your eyes.

MAKEUP BRUSHES

An investment in a good set of natural-bristle brushes—lip brush, blush brush, powder brush, eye shadow brush, and flat brush—will last a lifetime. Alternatively, you'll find great, sturdy natural-bristle brushes at bargain prices at an art supply store. Because they can harbor dust and bacteria that can cause breakouts, wash your brushes regularly with liquid soap or shampoo, and lay them out to air dry. Between cleanings, wipe them off with a tissue.

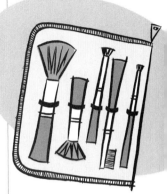

Look for soft brushes to deposit color evenly.

BIG BRUSH

Keep a powder brush handy, to sweep up excess makeup from your face.

BLOW-DRYER

To protect your hair and keep it soft and silky, let it air dry whenever possible. If you can't do this during the week, at least give it a break over the weekend. Always blow-dry on a low setting to protect your hair from heat damage.

BODY BRUSH

The skin on your body is thicker than the skin on your face, and it needs to be exfoliated, too. Buy a long-handled natural-bristle brush and brush your dry body before you step into the bath or shower, especially in the winter months. It sloughs off dead skin, increases circulation and leaves your skin feeling tingly and invigorated.

beauty to go

Before you head out into the great, wild world, here are the four
basic bits of beauty booty that it pays to tote with you

1 Concealer.
Instead of wearing foundation, you can simply use concealer to cover up blemishes and broken capillaries, along with other marks and discolorations. Look for a dual-palette concealer and mix the tones so that it blends in perfectly with your skin.

2 Color.
If you have a minimal makeup style, simply toss a tube of cheek gel and a pot of gloss in your bag. Or, if you really like to travel light, try multipurpose lip-and-cheek tints, which work particularly well if your makeup palette is neutral. (See page 233.)

3 Lip balm.
Everyone gets dry lips, and a smidge of moisturizing lip balm not only feels good, it can heal chapped lips. (It's also great for massaging into your cuticles and dabbing on dry patches of skin in a pinch.)

4 Mascara.
A flick of the mascara wand is quick and easy, it costs little, and the payoff is huge. Especially as we get older, the eye-popping power of mascara becomes harder to ignore.

TIP: *If you like the definition your lashes get from black mascara but not the harshness, try charcoal— a soft black— instead.*

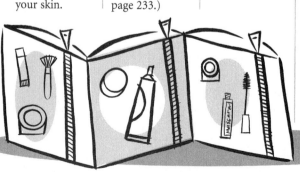

THE BEAUTY PANTRY

Just as a well-stocked kitchen pantry is lined with jars of grains, mustard, peanut butter, canned soup, and more, your beauty pantry should never be without these handy items—most of them basic household products. Whether it's a stash of waxing strips to catch that spot on your upper lip that the aesthetician missed or a bottle of lavender essential oil to apply to a kitchen stove burn, they'll prove invaluable when you need a quick fix. Most are amazing multitaskers that can substitute for other products in a pinch.

ALUM BLOCK

An alum block looks like a small piece of white quartz, although it's actually composed of potassium phosphate and alum (a mineral). This little piece of magic has many uses: as an underarm deodorant, an overnight zit-zapper, and as a way to stanch bleeding from shaving nicks.

BAKING SODA

Baking soda can be used to brush your teeth, applied as a paste to dry a pimple overnight, or massaged through damp hair to get rid of built-up styling products. Baking soda can also be rubbed on flaky elbows and knees and used as an exfoliant on the face.

AN OLD TOOTHBRUSH (AND TOOTHPASTE)

Like a cat, a toothbrush has many lives, and as an accessory to beauty, a recycled toothbrush is indispensable. Use it as a comb

BEAUTY CRUSADE

The Crusades were ostensibly fought over religion, but there's another, lesser-known reason: People were fighting over land rich in alum. In those days, alum was a cure-all for a variety of ailments.

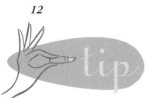

SUGAR SCRUB

Sweeten your bath or shower with a handful of sugar— brown or white— and use it as a body scrub. A sugar-and-water paste will also exfoliate dry, flaky skin or stubborn rough spots on elbows, knees, and heels.

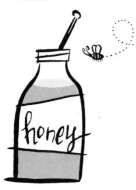

honey

for eyebrows and eyelashes; as an applicator for hair dye and touch-ups; as an exfoliator for lips, elbows, and knees; and as an all-purpose scrubber for beauty tools like pencil sharpeners, combs, and tweezers.

SWEET ALMOND OIL

This is my beauty panacea; it's a great moisturizer for dry skin, because it absorbs so neatly, and it's a handy eye makeup remover when you're without. It softens cuticles, makes dry hair supple and adds shine, and will also stand in for bath oil when your body needs softening. Buy a big bottle at the health-food store for $4.

HONEY

Honey is antibacterial, which makes it lovely to use on oily or blemished skin. (Cover a blemish with a dab of honey, place a Band-Aid over it, and it will be gone by morning.) Its stickiness makes it a terrific adhesive to hold ingredients together in face masks. In Vermont folk medicine traditions, honey is applied to a burn to relieve pain and prevent blisters. How sweet is that?

BABY WIPES

Not just for babies, these wipes will remove stubborn eye makeup in a pinch, as well as most lipstick and other makeup smudges from clothes. Gently pat the stain with the wipe and moisten with water. They'll also clean scuff marks from freshly polished toes that are exposed in sandals.

LAVENDER ESSENTIAL OIL

Even if you're not into the aromatherapy scene, keep one essential oil in the house—lavender. It has so many therapeutic uses: tip a few drops into the tub for a relaxing bath, keep it in the kitchen because nothing soothes a burn—and prevents blistering and scarring—like lavender oil, or massage on joints to relieve arthritis pain.

BATH SALTS

The ultimate, cost-efficient stress buster, a handful of sweet-smelling bath salts in a warm bath is relaxing, will lift your mood, and can also soothe tired muscles. Plus, if you massage the salts into your damp skin before you ease into the bath, your skin will more easily absorb moisturizer.

BAG OF FROZEN PEAS OR BLUEBERRIES

For pain and swelling in a bruised knee or ankle, for a burn, or for skin irritated by waxing, keep a bag of frozen fruit or veggies in the freezer. Their malleable shape adjusts easily around any part of your body.

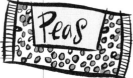

TEA BAGS

Keep black tea bags, green tea bags, and chamomile tea bags around the house for the many uses described throughout this book. Wet tea bags will help take down puffiness under the eyes and soothe bruises and mild burns. Chamomile soothes stressed

GLOBAL BRUSH-UP

Every culture has its own method of exfoliation. Coastal Europeans rub dried seaweed into their skin. Israelis massage with Dead Sea salts. Iranians use pulverized black volcanic rock. And Central Americans use the burlaplike fibers of the agave plant. In Japanese bathhouses, natural-bristle brushes are used to vigorously scrub the body from the neck down.

CLEAN UP YOUR ACT

Women have tremendous pack-rack potential, even when it comes to what we carry in our purses. Lighten your load. Go through your makeup bag and throw out anything old or that you never use. Get rid of stubby pencils, wash dirty brushes, and throw out bits of tissue and grubby sharpeners.

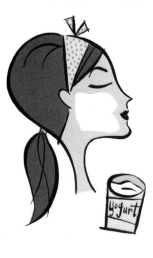

skin, and a chamomile compress will reduce irritation. After a bikini wax, for example, soak a cloth in warm chamomile tea and apply to skin for up to ten minutes.

CLAY MASK

Not only is a clay-based mask a great way to soak up excess oil from your face (and chest, and back), the clay also dries up pimples and soothes itchy insect bites.

COLD WAXING STRIPS

If you wax the hair on your face—whether you do it yourself or have it done professionally—you should lay in a stash of these. They are great for touch-ups, they'll extend your salon wax, and they'll curb the temptation to tweeze any stray hairs that sprout up uninvited on your face.

YOGURT

Plain low-fat (or nonfat) yogurt is not only good for you—calcium, ladies, calcium—it's good for your hair and skin. If you apply it to skin that feels tight and dry, it will soothe it, soften it, and make it feel silkier, too. Apply it to oily skin, and it will absorb excess oil. Massage yogurt into an itchy, flaky scalp, leave it on for 15 minutes, and rinse, and your flakes will be gone.

CHEESECLOTH

Great for wrapping bath soaks, poultices, sachets, and goopy face masks.

CHAPTER TWO

Fast Face

BVIOUSLY, NO ONE "NEEDS" MAKEUP, BUT WE'RE irresistibly drawn to those sleek, shiny pots and gorgeous, glittery pigments for good reason—they're pretty, they're pleasurable, and they hold out a promise. The attraction is almost as old as recorded history. In fact, a gold cosmetics kit was recently unearthed in an excavation from a Sumerian tomb dating back to the third millennium B.C.—the earliest evidence of makeup use.

Makeup appeals to our imagination and sense of play: With makeup, we can "play up" or "play down" whatever features we think are more or less attractive. A makeup artist once told me, "As much as women may complain about their looks, most don't want to look like anyone else." That's why it helps to learn a few easy, effortless techniques, enough to feel confident that you're putting your best face forward as you dash out the door. Putting on makeup doesn't demand a lot of time, and it offers immediate gratification. A little bit of color can effect subtle, beautiful changes—softer, fuller lips; healthy-looking, flushed cheeks; bigger, bolder eyes.

If you ask any woman how much time she wants to spend putting on her makeup, she'll probably tell you, "Five minutes or less." Well, you can accomplish a lot in five minutes. A natural or glamorous look can take anywhere from 30 seconds to 15 minutes, and as you become more practiced, you'll learn how to pare down your makeup regimen even further.

Get to know your face without makeup. Zero in on what you believe is your best feature, so that you can play it up. Some women have great eyes, lush lashes, a pretty mouth. Some have beautiful cheekbones. Focus.

No matter what your style—or, for that matter, your age or your mood—you'll want to streamline the process to get the most out of your makeup in as little time as possible. To learn to do less, but do it well, may take a bit of practice. So arm yourself with a bottle of makeup remover and set aside 30 minutes one evening to test out a few techniques that are highlighted in each of the sections below. These fast faces—from a low-key casual to a more elegant look—are guides that will help you look and feel more attractive and confident, without feeling like you're wearing a lot of makeup.

THE 30-SECOND Face

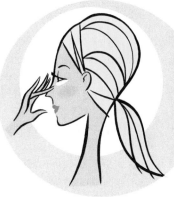

For those low-key "ponytail" days, when you're planning to stick close to home, run errands, spend the morning at the playground, or go to the gym, here's how to perk up a natural look with minimal effort and virtually no time. Remember, no matter how little time you have, always apply sun protection and moisturizer.

STEP 1 **CONCEALER** *(15 seconds)*

Dot cream concealer on blemishes and undereye circles. To apply a minimum of makeup quickly, use your fingers (use your fourth finger on the undereye area). The warmth of your finger helps the makeup "melt" into your skin.

PRODUCTS: Laura Mercier Undercover ▪ Stila Eye Concealer ▪ Nars Eye Brightener ▪ Philosophy the Supernatural Color Correctors.

STEP 2 **COLOR** *(5 seconds)*

Dab a tiny bit of liquid or gel blush on your cheeks and work it in with your fingers until there are no edges. Or, for a sun-kissed look, apply bronzing powder over cheekbones and browbones. Stroke on some lip gloss.

STEP 3 **HAIR** *(10 seconds)*

Slick your hair back and gather it into a coated elastic band. If you like, separate a piece of hair from the ponytail, wind it around the elastic to cover it, and tuck it into the elastic under the ponytail or fasten it with a bobby pin.

THE 2-MINUTE Face

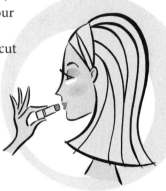

As long as you stick with a simple, efficient routine, you can get your makeup done in two minutes. I promise. Multipurpose products shortcut and streamline your regime because they accomplish more with less: less product, less expense, and, ultimately, less time before you're ready to run out the door. See "Beauty Products," pages 233–234, for more information.

STEP 1 **BASE** *(30 seconds)*

Apply tinted moisturizer or sheer foundation (SPF 15) all over your face, or wherever you feel you need coverage, like the shadows on the sides of your nose or red eyelids. Apply creamy concealer to the undereye area with your fourth finger and blend outward toward the sides of your face.

STEP 2 **COLOR** *(30 seconds)*

Using a dual cheek- and lip-tint product, apply color to the apples of your cheeks and your lips. Apply lip gloss for a hint of shine.

STEP 3 **EYELASH CURL** *(45 seconds)*

A quick turn with an eyelash curler or a stroke of curling mascara on the lash tips can provide an eye-opening shortcut.

STEP 4 **HAIR** *(15 seconds)*

After brushing your hair, give it instant shine. Use shine serum on thick hair, hair cream or light pomade on wavy or curly hair, and hair oil on fine hair.

TEST YOUR COLOR PALETTE

Everyone's skin tone breaks down into two color families: (1) *warm* has yellow undertones, and (2) *cool* has pink undertones. Once you determine your skin tone, you'll have a much easier time honing in on the most flattering makeup shades, which basically fall into the pink or peach family. Here are four easy ways to test for your skin tone.

▓ Try on a gold bracelet and a silver one. Which looks better? If it's gold, you're warm, and if it's silver, you're cool.

▓ Take something orange and something pink—like a scarf or a towel—and drape it around your head. If the pink looks better against your skin, you're cool; if the orange is more flattering, you're warm.

▓ Take a look at the veins on the inside of your wrist. Are they blue? Then you're cool. Are they greenish? You're warm.

▓ Try on a white top, then try on an off-white or cream-colored top. Does the cream look better? You're warm, so look for peachy tones. Does the white look better? You're cool, so pink shades look best on you.

THE 5-MINUTE FACE

It only takes five minutes to create a polished, pulled-together look. Whether you've got an important meeting, a lunch date, or a presentation at work, a few extra minutes will give you time to really even out your skin tone and focus on your eyes.

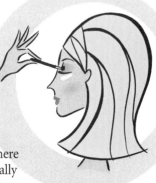

STEP 1 **SKIN** (*30 seconds*)

Apply concealer under the eyes and elsewhere on your face where you need it. Blend really well. Then apply foundation or tinted moisturizer. Now here's a little secret: Only use foundation where you need it—to even out your skin tone, to cover redness on either side of your nose, to cover blemishes or discoloration. The same holds true for powder. Apply a light dusting or brush it on only where you feel you need it—your nose, chin, or forehead.

STEP 2 EYE SHADOW *(1 minute)*

Sweep a light, neutral eye shadow all over your lids. Choose an innocuous shade that looks like it won't make any difference, such as sand, khaki, tawny, or beige. You're not making a color statement here; you're trying to neutralize any red in your lids and bring light to your eyes to make them pop. If you want something slightly more dramatic, smudge a medium to darker shade on the lids from the lash line to the crease with an eye shadow brush.

STEP 3 EYELINER *(1 minute)*

For a fast focus on your eyes, the trick is in the technique. Until you get the hang of it, a pencil is easier to work with than liquid liner.

1. Rest your elbows on the table to keep your hands steady.

2. Use a pencil with a soft, not sharp, point and make a series of dots, one next to the other, as close to the upper lash line as you can get. Work quickly. It's hard to control a continuous line, but a series of close-together dots create the same depth. (Think Georges Seurat and pointillism.) If you want, line the lower lids as well. To soften the line, smudge with your finger, a small brush, or a hard-pressed Q-tip.

STEP 3 LIPS *(30 seconds)*

Color in your entire lip with a pencil and top with gloss from a pot or tube, or simply slide on gloss or lipstick.

STEP 4 CHEEKS *(30 seconds)*

Apply a sheer pink or peach blush on the apples of your cheeks and blend well. Make sure the edges are blended so there are no harsh lines of demarcation.

ONE GREAT TOOL: THE EYELASH CURLER

I eschewed the eyelash curler for way too long, until I looked in the mirror one day and realized that my eyelashes seemed to be getting straighter as I got older. My eyes were disappearing into my head, and I had to do something! Et, voila! A gift was sent to my office from the French beauty goddesses—a Talika Heated Eyelash Curler. I tried it—in the right sequence, after I applied SPF-tinted moisturizer and before I put in my contact lenses. Then I put on my mascara. I'm telling you, the curler has really opened my eyes. They look bigger, fresher, saucier! And my mascara never smudges anymore, since my lashes have become so perky.

TIP: *If you've already got an eyelash curler but it's not self-heating, give it a quick blast with your blow-dryer to heat it up before you use it.*

STEP 5 **LASHES** *(1 minute)*

Curl your lashes and coat them with mascara.

STEP 6 **HAIR LIFT** *(30 seconds)*

To give curly hair a morning lift, turn your head upside down, spray some volumizer at the roots, scrunch your fingers through, turn right-side up, and smooth it down. If your hair is straight or wavy, apply a bit of volumizer to your fingers, massage it into the roots, lifting the hair as you go, and gently pat it through your hair to give it a sleeker finish.

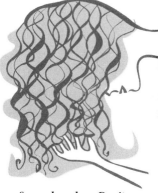

Scrunch and go. Don't manipulate curly hair too much or it turns to frizz.

PRODUCTS: John Sahag Air Lift ■ Phyto Phytovolume Actif Maximizing Volume Spray for Fine and Limp Hair ■ Aussie Real Volume Leave-In Volumizer.

foolproof mascara

Start by applying mascara only to the top lashes. That may be enough—especially if you're prone to smudging. If you like to wear it on both the top and bottom fringe, apply it to your bottom lashes first.

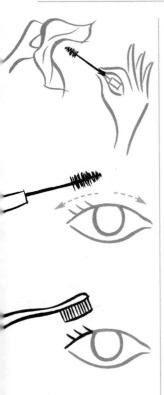

1 First, wipe off the mascara wand with a tissue or against the sides of the tube so that the mascara won't clump on your lashes.

2 Roll out the wand on your lashes from the base to the ends. Start with the middle lashes, then apply to the lashes on each side.

3 Let one coat dry for abut 30 seconds, then apply another.

4 After you apply, brush through your lashes with an old toothbrush or an eyelash comb.

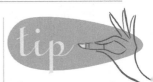

tip

If you want to make your eyes look like they're set farther apart, apply the mascara slightly diagonally and outward, toward the outer corners of your eyes.

EYESHADOW SHADES

Choosing the best eye shadow shade seems to be one of the most mystifying color choices for many women. The first thing to consider when choosing an eye shadow is how to enhance your eye color. Here are some basic guidelines about which colors go with which eye colors to help narrow down your options.

Brown Eyes: Shades of green, bronze, copper, amber, pale blue, and gold will create subtle drama that will deepen the color of your eyes.

Blue or Gray Eyes: Shades with hints of brown (i.e., brick, peach, purple) or yellow-gold, apricot, or copper bring out the blue or smokey gray.

Hazel or Green Eyes: Mauve, gold, pale purple, pewter, lilac, bronze, light brown, apricot, and khaki will make those gold and green lights flicker.

THE 15-MINUTE FACE

Day into Night

Evening is a great time to play around with deeper lip shades—like red, garnet, and burgundy—and sexy, smoky shadow on the eyes, because these rich tones work well with soft, evening lighting. If you harbor a secret desire to wear red lipstick, but can't work up the nerve, experiment with a lighter, sheerer texture—for example, instead of a matte or creamy red lipstick, try red lip gloss.

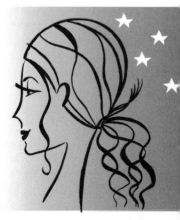

When you're going out for the evening or prepping for a special event, you may want to build in a few

extra minutes to get ready—but you don't need any more than
15, and less than 10 if you skip the first step or two in the game
plan below.

STEP 1 **BROWS** *(3 minutes)*

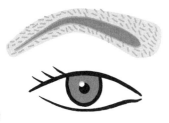

"With the right arch," a makeup
artist once told me, "you can
tell right away that a woman feels sexy."
There is, truly, a sophisticated insou-
ciance about a well-shaped brow. Here
are a few foolproof hints that will help
you avoid common plucking pitfalls like
spotty or overarching brows.

Before you tweeze, design the shape you want by filling in your
brows with eye shadow. Think of the hairs as if they grew in horizontal rows, and tweeze a single horizontal row at a time. Stop often,
stand back, and look in the mirror to see how you're doing. Make
sure to stop while you're ahead—that last hair you're going for is
always the one you should leave alone.

Groom your brows with a brow brush, if needed, to shape them
and help them lie flat.

STEP 2 **FACE MASK** *(5 minutes)*

A quick mask before a night out can give your skin an immediate
boost. It will also calm down any redness from tweezing. To
tighten the look of your skin, try a *firming mask*. To absorb excess
oil and make your pores look smaller, use a *clay mask* with kaolin
or bentonite. To plump up your skin and suffuse it with a glow, try
a *moisturizing mask*.

Apply the mask, lie down for 5 minutes, elevate your legs, and
take some deep, slow belly breaths. Rinse with cool water.

PRODUCTS: Naturopathica Environmental Defense Mask ▪ Yves Rocher Hydrating Mask
with Mallow Extract ▪ Eau Thermale Avene Instant Soothing Moisture Mask ▪ Boscia Moisture
Replenishing Mask ▪ Clinique Anti-Gravity Firming Lift Mask ▪ Benefit Cosmetics Hi Neighbor!
Friendly Face Mask ▪ Osea White Algae Mask for sensitive skin.

STEP 3 **SKIN** *(30 seconds)*

Apply foundation or concealer where needed. Try a light-reflecting foundation if you want a look that's less matte and more luminous. Here's the fun part: Try "light-diffusing" or "light-reflecting" makeup—it's sheer and contains tiny bits of pulverized minerals that catch and reflect the light. It literally lights up your face and gives it a glow.

STEP 4 **EYE SHADOW** *(2 minutes)*

To glam it up, try a smoky or shimmery eye shade. But if you do, keep the rest of your makeup fairly low-key.

"Pair high-drama eyes with natural lips and cheeks for the ultimate in sexy," says Jean Ford, cocreator and cofounder of Benefit Cosmetics, who offers these quick tips on how to achieve it:

Use an eye shadow brush to sweep a deep eye shadow shade (brown, gray, or purple) over the eyelid from lash line to crease. (Or, if you prefer, sweep a shimmery eye shadow shade from the lash line up toward your brows.)

Use a soft, black kohl pencil or eyeliner to line around the eye (see page 20). For a softer look—or if your coloring is medium to fair—try a brown pencil and smudge it slightly with a hard-pressed Q-tip or your finger to extend the eyes in the outer corners.

STEP 5 **MASCARA** *(1 minute)*

Curl your lashes and finish with a coat (or two) of mascara.

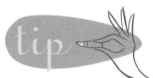

CALLING ALL BRUNETTES

I picked up this great tip from makeup artist Bobbi Brown: If you're a brunette, always keep a mahogany shade of eye shadow handy. You can use it— along with a small makeup brush or old toothbrush—to fill in spotty brows, line your eyes, and cover gray roots along your hairline between touch-ups.

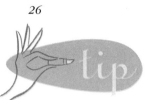

LIP TIPS

A lip brush gives you more precision. When you apply lip color directly from the tube—or with fingers—it's a softer look. After applying lipstick, pull your finger through the puckered "O" in your lips to prevent lipstick on your teeth.

STEP 6 **COLOR** *(90 seconds)*

Dab a bit of blush on your cheeks and blend. If your lipstick tends to feather or bleed, outline your lips first with a nude lip pencil. For more definition on your lips—especially if you're wearing a deep shade like burgundy or red—apply the lip color with a brush. When you use a lip brush, blend the lipstick toward the middle of the mouth to prevent a "ring" of lipstick at the edges.

STEP 7 **POWDER** *(30 seconds)*

Dust on a light coat of translucent powder, but keep it light. Too much powder can settle into lines and creases, making the skin look dry and crepey.

STEP 8 **CHIC HAIR** *(90 seconds)*

If you don't have time to wash your hair, good! Unwashed hair actually holds a style better. Slick your hair back, make a low- to mid-level ponytail, twist a piece of hair around the base, and tuck the ends in. (If necessary, secure with bobby pins.) If you like a looser, more casual look, pull a few strands out or scrunch your fingers through to loosen the do. A side benefit to wearing your hair pulled back is that it puts more emphasis on your face.

SOMETHING FESTIVE

Colored mascara may sound scary, but it's a great way to liven up your party look in 2 seconds flat. First, apply a coat of black or brown mascara to the lashes. Then lightly tip the ends with burgundy (for blue eyes) or blue or green (for brown eyes) to make your peepers pop.

day into night fast fix

I f you have to go out right after work and only have two minutes to make the transition, simply build on the makeup you've worn during the day.

1 **Moisturize**.

2 **Touch up** your concealer.

3 **Refresh** the color on your cheeks.

4 **Reapply** your eyeliner or eye shadow, or layer a shimmer shadow on top of the one you're already wearing. For example, if you're wearing a tawny brown eye shadow, a sweep of bronze shimmer shadow will add sparkle to your eyes.

5 **Use** a big, pouffy brush to dust on a sprinkling of powder wherever your face gets shiny. To help your cheekbones stand out, apply a bit of shimmer powder to the apples of your cheeks.)

6 **Touch up** the tips of your lashes with mascara.

7 **Glide on** lip gloss, and go!

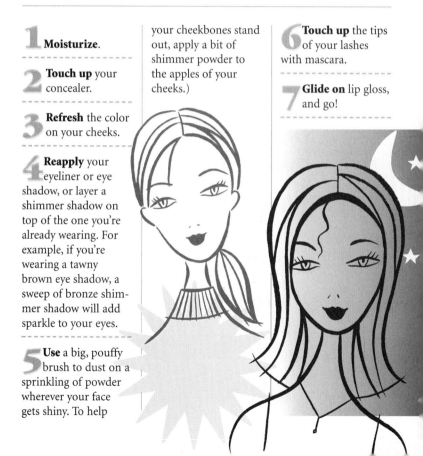

THE ART OF ILLUSION

W omen have always depended on tricks to tweak reality a bit—creating the appearance of bigger eyes, lusher lips, a smaller nose, higher cheekbones, and smooth, unmarked skin—and they probably always will.

Nothing looks as good as naturally healthy skin, but let's be honest. We all have moments when we want to fake it: to cover up or "correct" perceived flaws, to enhance what nature may— or may not—have given us. In this section, I'll show you how a little sleight of hand—like a judicious swipe of cosmetic color— can create the desired illusion.

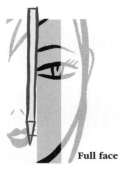

Full face

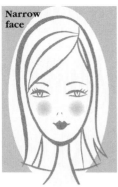

Narrow face

Face Fixes

FULL FACE

A strong arch in your brows can de-emphasize the fullness in your face. Hold a pencil vertically alongside your nose. Your brows should start where the nose side of the pencil meets your browline. Now, place the eraser end of the pencil along your outer iris. Your arch should peak to where the top of the pencil points. Proceed slowly—only tweeze a couple of hairs at a time, then check the mirror—to avoid pencil-thin or round brows.

NARROW FACE

If your face is long and narrow, like Sarah Jessica Parker's, apply blush to the apples of your cheeks, not out to the temples, or it will make your face look longer.

SQUARE FACE

To soften the shape, apply blush to the apples of your cheeks, and fan it out to your temples.

WIDE FACE

Apply blush only on the apples of your cheeks, but don't go too close to your nose, and don't fan the color out to your ears, or it will make your wide face look wider.

DOUBLE CHIN

This takes a bit of practice, but if you want to camouflage a double chin, brush a bit of rose-brown blush along your jaw from your earlobes to your chin. Highlight your chin with light translucent powder. Make sure to blend really, really well.

FINE LINE ERASERS

Makeup that contains light-reflecting particles can reflect light away from your lines and make them appear to disappear. Apply it all over your face, or under the eyes or on laugh lines.

PRODUCTS: L'Oréal Translucide Lasting Luminous Makeup ▪ Lancôme Photogenic Ultra Comfort ▪ Prescriptives Luxe Softglow Moisture Makeup ▪ Clinique Dewy Smooth Anti-Aging Makeup SPF 15.

DEEP LINE ERASERS

Let's say you wake up one morning and the lines on your forehead, or between

HISTORICAL FAKE-OUTS

In the Victorian era, it was officially frowned upon for women to wear makeup, but the clever beauty mavens of the day found other ways to flush their cheeks, redden their lips, and give their eyes that era's fashionably limpid look. Victorian women were advised to pinch their cheeks, bite their lips, and grate horseradish into cold milk and apply it to the skin to improve its color. One bit of folklore said to rub cheeks with a crimson silk cloth dipped in wine. (Of course, if you rubbed hard enough, your cheeks would flush, regardless of the color of the cloth—or the wine.)

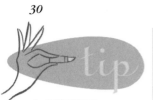

A LITTLE DAB'LL DO YA

To make your cheekbones really stand out, take a slightly darker shade of blush—a light brown or tan—and dab a tiny bit in the hollows of your cheeks, under the bones. Use only a tiny bit and blend well.

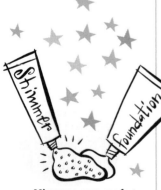

Mix your own made-to-order, perfect product

your nose and mouth, look deeper than usual. Do what 40-plus models and celebs do when prepping for a photo shoot: Reach for the cosmetic spackle—no kidding—and fill them in.

PRODUCTS: Prescriptives Invisible Line Smoother ■ Clinique Line Smoothing Concealer.

LOFTY FOREHEAD

To make a high forehead look less lofty, take a matte powder bronzer or blush that's a shade darker than your foundation and brush it along your hairline, from above your ears to the middle of your forehead. Blend well, brushing toward your hair.

GREAT CHEEKBONES

Using a powder blush, stroke blush upward, once, on the apples of your cheeks, toward your ears, then go back over it in a choppy, up-and-down movement.

GET GLOWING

Mix your foundation or tinted moisturizer with a luminizer or illuminating moisturizer or, when the lights are low and you want to glow, try a foundation with a bit of shimmer. Don't be afraid of shimmer products; they're like the outfit that doesn't look like much when it's on the hanger, but looks great once you put it on!

PRODUCTS: Lorac Oil-Free Luminizer ■ Prescriptives Vibrant Vitamin Infuser for Dull, Stressed Skin.

FREEBIES: BEFORE YOU BUY, TRY

If you want to update your look, make a change, or simply pick up a few new ideas, stop at the cosmetics counter for some expert help. But try before you buy. Many cosmetics companies—including high-end brands like Chanel, Clarins, and Clinique—are quite generous with their give-aways. With smaller companies, you may be able to find a sample- or travel-size portion to try before making too much of an investment. (See pages 248–249 for Web sites that offer free samples and discounts.)

And, of course, there's always Sephora—a beauty playland where you're encouraged to, literally, stick your Q-tip in every pot. Note: Make sure to swab the sampler with a tissue or cotton pad first to remove the top layer before you apply it to your face.

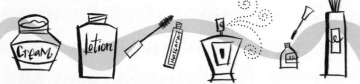

Here are a few tips when you go to the makeup counter:

■ Don't go to the makeup counter when your skin is acting up. The advice you get will be directed toward skincare and makeup that offers coverage, and if your skin is usually in good shape, those products are not what you need.

■ Look for a salesperson whose makeup style is one you like and whose coloring is similar to yours.

■ Go when the store is less crowded (say, weekday mornings), and you'll get more time and attention.

■ Be specific and tell the makeup artist what you like and dislike and how much time you're willing to spend on your makeup. If you know you're not going to take the time to apply two shades of eye shadow, say so.

■ Bring makeup-remover cloths or baby wipes so that you can wipe it off in the ladies' room if you don't like it.

■ Remember, you don't *need* to buy anything unless you *want* to. And you don't need to buy the whole "program." Mixing cosmetic brands is as good an idea as mixing clothing designers.

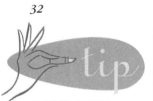

SOFT SKIN

*If your foundation
or tinted moisturizer
tend to look too dry
on your face, mix
them with a dab of
moisturizer before
you apply.*

DON'T KNOW WHERE THE YELLOW WENT!

On those days when you wake up looking jaundiced, a single, all-around application of sheer pinkish powder will warm up your face and neutralize the yellow tones. The key is to look for a shade that's sheer, so that you will see the warming effect of the color, not the color itself.

PRODUCTS: Nars Blush in Orgasm ■ Benefit Cosmetics Dandelion.

BLAH DAY

When your skin just looks blah, try a lotion with pinkish undertones to give it some radiance. But not too much—apply to cheeks and browbones only—or you'll look too shiny.

PRODUCTS: Laboratoire Remède Soft Focusing Lotion ■ Benefit Cosmetics Hollywood Glo ■ American Beauty Luminous Liquid All-Over Face Glow (Pink).

SLIMMING HAIR STYLES

If you're on a weight-loss program, but you're not yet where you want to be, here are some dos and don'ts to flatter a full face:

Yes. Long, sleek lines around the face will de-emphasize fullness. Try highlights or lowlights around the face, a hair length that's between the jaw line and the shoulders, a side part, or an updo style.

No. Extreme lengths and extreme shapes will make your face look fuller. Avoid really long, really short, really big, really curly or wedge-shaped cuts. Try to avoid too much hair at the sides of your face and by your ears.

ONE-SIDED BREAKOUTS

If you break out on one side of your face more than the other, it's probably your phone side, where bacteria on your phone is pressed into your skin all day. Wipe your phone daily with an antibacterial cleanser and alternate ears. While we're on the subject, change your pillowcases often—a dirty pillowcase is another cause of breakouts.

STAYING POWDER

Powder blush will give you a nice, matte finish, and cream blush will give your cheeks a glow, but they don't always have great staying power, especially if your skin is oily. For long-lasting color on your cheeks, try liquid blush or cheek gel.

PRODUCTS: M·A·C Cheekhue ■ Bliss Ink Pink Blushing Balm ■ Vincent Longo Cheek Gel ■ Napoleon Barely Blushing Cheek Gel.

THE EYES

The best eye makeup is almost imperceptible, yet it brightens your eyes, enhances their shape, and makes them look more expressive.

CLOSE-SET EYES

To create the illusion of more space between your eyes, emphasize the outer corners with makeup and concentrate your efforts away from the center. Apply light eye shadow from the inner corner to the iris and

BUFF PUFF

Try this makeup artist's tip at home: Go back and forth over your face with a clean drugstore powder puff to buff your face powder and matte it out so your face won't look too shiny, or too powdery, either.

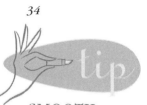

SMOOTH OPERATOR

To avoid clumps when you apply mascara, wiggle the wand from side to side from the base of your lashes to the tips.

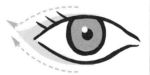

After outlining eyes, gently smudge with fingers for a soft, sexy look.

darker shadow from the iris out toward the edges. Blend well. Using a pencil or kohl crayon, draw a line (see page 20) as close to the lash line as possible, from the outer edge of the iris to the outer corners of your top and bottom lash lines. Smudge slightly with fingers or a hard-pressed Q-tip.

WIDE-SET EYES

To make eyes look closer together, apply a bit of dark liner on the inner corners of your eyes and blend. If you wear eye shadow, apply it starting at the inner corner of the eye, but let it fade out before the outer edges.

DEEP-SET EYES

Light colors come forward, and dark colors recede. To bring your eyes forward, sweep a light shade of eye shadow on your lids, from the lashes to the brow. Don't use too much—it should be barely perceptible.

EYES LIKE SAUCERS

To elongate your eyes, line the outer two-thirds of your upper and lower lash lines, then join the lines at the outer corners of your eyes, turning up just a tiny bit. Apply mascara to the outer lashes only.

DROOPY EYES

Line the top lid along the lash line, pulling the line up slightly at the outer corners. Apply eye shadow on top of the line or smudge it to make it look softer.

EYES LIKE SLITS

To make your eyes look more open, curl lashes with an eyelash curler and apply mascara first to the middle lashes, then apply it on a diagonal toward the outer corners of your eyes.

PRODUCTS: Lancôme Hypnose Custom Volume Mascara ■ Bourjois Pump Up the Volume ■ Shu Uemura Mascara Basic ■ Hourglass Fiction Defining Mascara.

LIGHT LASHES

Have them tinted or line your eyes with brown pencil and stroke brown mascara on your lashes. If your brows are really light, black mascara can look too harsh.

THINNING BROWS

Whether your brows are thinning or starting to "pale out" with the growth of a few grays, you can make them look thicker in two ways: (1) Have your hairstylist or colorist tint them; (2) brush eye shadow or mascara on brows in a shade that matches your brow color (use a small flat brush for shadow), and comb it through with an eyebrow comb or clean mascara spoolie.

UNRULY BROWS

When some brow hairs grow in longer than others, just give them a trim. Brush your eyebrows northward with a brow brush or an old toothbrush. Trim any hairs that extend above the brow line with tiny scissors.

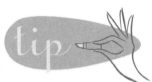

EYE OPENER

A subtle way to make your eyes look bigger is to apply a second coat of mascara only at the outer corners of your upper lashes.

SPOTTY BROWS

Fill in any gaps with a brow pencil, eye shadow, or eyebrow powder in the same color as your brows—or experiment with one shade lighter—and gently blend with your index finger or a small, flat brush.

BUSHY BROWS

If your brows go wild after a few hours, set them in place with a brow brush sprayed with a bit of hairspray or slick on a clear brow gel (or a dab of Vaseline), and brush them up and into shape.

PRODUCTS: Cover Girl Natural Lash ▪ Brow Mascara (a clear mascara).

BLONDIE BROWS

To give blond brows more oomph, apply eyebrow powder in a shade slightly darker than your brow color. Take a bit of the powder on an angled brush, shake it to remove the excess, and stroke it very lightly and gently over the brows in an outward direction. If you can't find your color in an eyebrow powder—Maybelline has a good range of colors—substitute a matte eye shadow in a shade slightly darker than your brows.

WEAK BROWS

Take a small, damp eye shadow brush or makeup sponge. Dip it into taupe, brown, or black eye shadow (whichever blends with your brow color), tap it to get

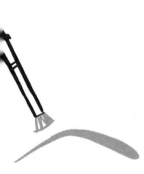

Brow pencils have more staying power, but powder creates a more natural look.

rid of any excess, and smooth a bit onto your brows. Or, after you've applied mascara, without redipping the wand, skim it over your brows, then blend with a small brush or toothbrush.

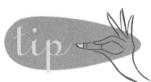

BEST BROWS

BROWS IN LIMBO

If you're in limbo waiting for your brows to grow in, dab cream concealer on stray hairs to cover them. To help define brows, use a brow wax. Use eye shadow or a pencil to fill in spotty regrowth, but don't add too much color and use a spoolie or a baby toothbrush to blend and soften it. Avoid shimmery eyeshadow while your brows grow in.

PRODUCTS: Benefit Cosmetics Brow Zing ▪ Lorac Brow Wax ▪ Laura Mercier Eyebrow Pencils ▪ M·A·C Eye Brows.

If you have no artistic talent when it comes to brow shaping, get them done by a makeup artist at a salon. Then, ask her to show you how you can maintain them at home.

WHITER WHITES

Sand-colored eye shadow is a neutral, understated shade that will make your eyes look less red. And yellow, believe it or not, can make the whites of the eyes look whiter. If your eyes are blue, try pale, lemony tones; if your eyes are dark, try yolky, custardy tones. Stroke over your lids with an eye shadow brush.

DELICATE LASHES

If your lashes are delicate, avoid mascara with thick-brush wands. Try a brand with a thin, short-bristle wand or comb; it will help your lashes look more naturally fuller without overwhelming your eyes.

RED HOT

Red is a hot, glamorous color, and, according to celebrity makeup artist Julie Hewett, "Almost anyone can wear some shade of red on her lips. It's a 2-second way to warm up your face." If you want to mute or tone down the intensity of red, apply lip balm first, layer red lipstick or a red lip pencil on top, then blot with paper until you get a stain. Or, apply lip pencil on top of lipstick.

THE LIPS

No cosmetic has the potential to punctuate your mood or express your personality like lipstick. For some women, a matte red lipstick may feel too flamboyant. For others, a clear, shiny gloss may be too sexual. For you, it may be just right. The lipstick shade and texture, as well as the technique you use, have the power to transform the shape and emphasis of your lips. Here are some lip lessons in illusion.

LIP PLUMPER

Moisten a bit of cinnamon and rub it on your lips before you apply lipstick. Or apply a bit of cinnamon oil to your lips (use only a drop as some people are sensitive to it). Or try lip plumpers with niacin, a form of vitamin B that pumps up the circulation and so plumps up the lips.

PRODUCTS: Alex and Ani Serious Lip Plump ▪ Freeze 24/7 Plump Lips ▪ Hydroderm Lip Plumper.

THIN LIPS

Apply a nude lip pencil to the center of the lower edge of the bottom lip or use an opalescent lipstick to create a fuller look.

OLD COLOR

Too much lip color can be aging, no matter how young you are. For a fresh look, give your lips a stain: Rub a lip brush against your lip pencil and then brush the color on your lips. Press it in with your finger.

WASHED OUT

Intense color on the lips will perk up your entire face. When you're feeling washed out and wan, it's time to slide a tube of red or garnet lipstick (or gloss) across your lips.

BLEEDING LIPSTICK

If you have oily skin, your lipstick may tend to bleed off your lips. Here are some correctives: Color in your lips before applying lipstick or gloss; outline your lips with a nude pencil (one that's dry, not creamy); or use a concealer pencil to fill in the lines around your lips and blend well.

LIPS ON THE DOWNTURN

Focus attention on the center of your mouth with a dab of gloss, and don't extend your lip color all the way out to the corners.

PEARLY WHITES

Your teeth deserve the same kind of TLC that you invest in your makeup and skincare regimens. A good set of pretty white teeth can really brighten up your look. Brush and floss at least twice a day (or after every meal), and do a spot check for stains on a regular basis.

FRESH MOUTH

If you can, try to brush your teeth after drinking tea, coffee, or red wine to prevent stains before they set.

My favorite lipstick shade has been discontinued. Is there anything I can do?

Two companies that specialize in custom blending—Giella and Three Custom Color Specialists—will take anything from an old lipstick to a piece of wallpaper (!) and match the color. Prescriptives does it, too, in select areas around the country.

CHAPTER THREE

BEAUTY MELTDOWNS

EVERY WOMAN WILL PROBABLY RECOGNIZE HERSELF in one of these scenes: Your friends are picking you up for a day at the beach, you've decided it's time to wax your own legs, but you're stuck on the side of the tub trying to get up the nerve to rip off the wax. You've got a meeting at your son's school, and your hair is hopelessly entangled in your hairbrush. You're running late to work, you've just put the finishing touches on your makeup, and your mascara smudges. And you feel as frustrated and helpless as a three-year-old. It's a Beauty Meltdown moment.

This chapter offers quick solutions for those beauty bloopers that catch us all off guard, usually at the worst possible moment. Don't stress! Thirty seconds are sometimes all that you need to plan and execute a stunningly fast—and brilliantly effective—fix.

THE Face

We've all been through it. The early-morning frenzy that results in a streak of mascara on your upper eyelids as you're running out of the house. That moment when you catch a glimpse of yourself in the car mirror and realize your blush could easily land you in center ring at the circus. The late afternoon shine that's reflecting from your face. Technology and technique come to the rescue!

SPLOTCHY MAKEUP

To remove smudges or splotches on your face without redoing your makeup, take a flat Q-tip, dip it into your moisturizer, and apply it to the splotch. Gone in an instant! Use the other side of the Q-tip to mop it up or smooth it out.

CLOWN FACE

You overdid your blush and you don't have time to wash it off. If you've applied too much powder blush, go over it with a clean brush to remove excess. To tone down cream or gel blush, apply a dab of moisturizer or tinted moisturizer to your cheeks.

FULLER BRUSH

You look at yourself in the side-view mirror on the way to work and can't believe how much makeup you've got on. Take a clean, medium- to large-size brush—the size of a powder or blush brush—and gently brush over your face. Wipe with a tissue, and brush again. The brush will pick up extra powder, foundation, and eye color, softening your look. If you don't have a brush handy, use the sponge from your compact.

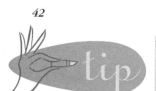

LIP LOSS

If your gloss slips off your lips in an hour, premix it with lipstick first on the back of your hand and use your index finger or a lip brush to apply it to your lips.

MAKEUP BLOOPER CHECKLIST

Before you head out the door, check your makeup in a mirror by a window in natural light for these common—but embarrassing—beauty blunders:

☐ Is your foundation blended above your lips, by the sides of your nose, and in front of your ears?

☐ Is there a rigid line of demarcation at your jaw that a field general could use to line up his troops?

☐ Is there foundation or powder on your eyebrows and grazing your hairline?

☐ Does your blush look like spots or stripes of color on your cheeks?

☐ Does the color splotch in front of your ears?

☐ Is your lipstick bleeding?

☐ Is there lipstick on your teeth?

☐ Is your mascara smudgy?

☐ Are your eyebrows disheveled and wild as weeds?

☐ Are there lines of concealer in the creases of your eyelids or undereyes?

SLIPPERY GLOSS

Gloss makes lips look juicy and healthy, but it doesn't have great staying power. For longer-lasting shine, first color in the lips with a nude pencil—the same color as your lips—and use a finger or a lip brush to blend the color into your lips like a stain. Then apply gloss on top.

CAKEY FACE

If your foundation looks cakey, spray your face lightly with water. Smooth out the edges with a damp sponge. Blend well.

SUPER STAIN

There is a type of super gloss that seems to survive through almost anything. Condition your lips first with lip balm, then apply one of the glosses below—they last longer and shine brighter, though they are stickier than average.

PRODUCTS: Clinique Color Surge Impossibly Glossy ▪ Estée Lauder Pure Color Lip Vinyl Gloss Stick ▪ Dior Addict Lip Fluid ▪ Bourjois Rouge Pop Chic ▪ M·A·C Lipglass.

LASTING LIPSTICK

Your lipstick will last through a three-course dinner if you powder your lips, apply lipstick, and blot it down with paper until the color stains the lips. Or, line your lips with pencil *after* you apply your lipstick.

LIP STAINS

Certain lip shades, especially heavy pigments, can be hard to remove. In a pinch, use your eye-makeup remover, then wash your lips. Or use sweet almond oil.

GUNKY MASCARA

Put your closed tube of mascara in a glass of hot water (submerge only ⅓ of the tube) for a minute or two. This will soften it so that it won't clump.

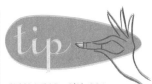

PENCIL IT IN

The drugstore brand Wet 'N Wild lip pencil #666 is a favorite of top makeup artists—and it only costs 99 cents!!

I love my creamy eye shadow but it always creases. What can I do?

Brush a shimmery translucent powder in a pale shade on top. It will keep the shadow where it belongs and light up your eyes—just make sure the powder isn't *too* iridescent or shimmery.

TUG O' WAR

If your lip pencil is so dry that it tugs across your skin, rub the tip between your fingers before you apply. Your body heat will soften it up just enough so that the color slides right on.

SIGHT LINES

Oily skin can make your eyeliner smudge. Liquid liner smudges least, but it's hardest to control. Try a dry compact liner, put it on wet with a liner brush, let it dry, and go over it with powder to prevent smudging. If you prefer a pencil, use a little brush to go over the line with matching eyeshadow to seal it.

LOWER LID SMUDGE

Lower lashes smudge more easily than the upper ones do, so if you're prone to smudge, leave your bottom lashes bare. But if you must, here's a foolproof tip: Wipe your wand with a tissue and, holding the wand *vertically*, go back and forth from inner to outer corners of your lower lashes. Take a thin, dry sponge and dab translucent powder up close to the lash line.

THE CRYING GAME

A crying jag at work smudged your mascara. Put a dab of makeup remover or toner on a Q-tip, and wipe it off. Or carry a portable product like Swabplus Waterproof Mascara Remover Swabs in your purse—until you find a new job!

TIRED EYES

A bit of eyeliner in a light shade will make tired eyes look brighter. The classic remedy is to line the inside of your lid with a white pencil, but this can look harsh. Try a peachy pink shade instead—it looks warmer and more natural. In some women, however, it can make your eyes look pinker—so be warned!

PRODUCT: Paula Dorf Baby Eyes Enhancer.

HARD LINE

If you want to smudge the line around your eyes to make it look softer, use hard-pressed Q-tips, or try the Laura Mercier smudge brush.

BABY RACCOON

Even if you don't get dark circles under your eyes, there's bound to come a night that results in dark shadows under your eyes in the morning. Mix a dab of undereye concealer in your palm with a bit of eye cream, and pat around the undereye area.

PRODUCTS: Benefit Cosmetics Eye Con ▪ La Mer The Eye Balm ▪ Olay Total Effects Eye Cream ▪ L'Oréal Visible Lift Eye Line-Minimizing Concealer.

FLAKING OFF

Sometimes dry, flaky patches won't respond to your usual moisturizer. Before you call your dermatologist, apply a thin layer of Kraft Miracle Whip to the spot. Leave on for about

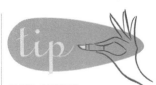

LIP LUBE

Fat lip pencils and chubby crayons are softer and less drying than regular, slim pencils.

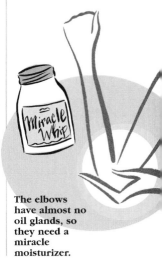

The elbows have almost no oil glands, so they need a miracle moisturizer.

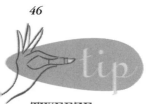

TWEEZE PLEASE

A slanted tweezer like Tweezerman or Rubis grabs really well. Once you become proficient, you may want to invest in a pointed tweezer, the tool of experts.

ten minutes, then gently massage the skin. Rinse with warm water and moisturize.

SNOWY BROWS

Brush away the flakes with an old toothbrush. Gently massage face oil into the brows. (Even a dab of olive or canola oil will soothe flakes.)

PRODUCTS: Ole Henriksen Black Currant Energizing Complexion Oil ■ Aveeno Creamy Moisturizing Oil.

OVERPLUCKED LIKE A CHICKEN

You've overdone it, and your brows look mangy and thin. Take an eye pencil (the same color as, or one shade lighter than, your brows), warm the tip between your fingers, and lightly fill in your brows, moving the strokes out toward the ears. You can also use eye shadow powder for the job. (Powder looks softer, but pencil has more staying power.) Brush on the brow hairs with a small, slanted brush in quick outward strokes, and blend with a dry mascara spoolie. Gently brush the brows with a brow brush to remove excess.

PALE FACE

You catch a glimpse of yourself in a mirror at work and find your pallor positively ghostly. To warm up your face, dip a brush in a powder blush (shake to remove excess) and apply a light dusting all over your face. This works well with bronzing powder, too, though most women are more likely to have blush handy.

SUPER NATURAL COLOR

A facial will get your glow going, but if you don't have time, mash a few strawberries in a nonreactive bowl and brush on clean skin with a pastry brush. Leave on for five minutes—you'll feel a slight tingling as the natural fruit acids in the berries start to rev up your circulation and exfoliate dead skin—and rinse with warm, then cool water.

MORNING-AFTER BEARD BURN

It was a fun night, but . . . Massage a tiny dab of over-the-counter cortisone cream into your skin. It should take the redness down, pronto!

STIFF UPPER LIP

You've waxed, and your upper lip is irritated. Be careful—some moisturizers will make it worse. Instead, apply sweet almond oil to the spot. Then apply a bag of frozen peas or blueberries to the lip area for a few minutes until the redness calms down.

POST-PARTY POOPERS

Some women find that their face breaks out after a night on the town. Drink lots of water throughout the evening and during the day to keep yourself hydrated. Make sure to wash off your makeup before you fall into bed, and put some prophylactic acne medication on those areas usually prone to breakouts.

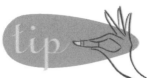

MORE IS LESS

Most of the time, when we try to hide something with powder, we end up highlighting it instead. Wipe your powder brush with a tissue and use it to go back over your face to pick up and remove any excess powder.

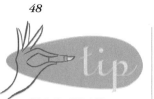

TOO-FLAT MATTE

This is a great tip for an evening out: If you love your lipstick, but the color looks flat and matte and not festive enough, dab a spot of shimmer eye shadow in the middle of your lower lip.

SPOT ON

If you—or your facialist—has busted a blemish, and you've got a red spot on your face, apply Neosporin Original First Aid Antibiotic Ointment before you go to bed. It will take down the redness and the spot overnight.

GET THE RED OUT

If you wake up with a pimple, Visine will take the red out. Apply a dab to the blemish. Then, using a small brush, stroke a bit of oil-free concealer in a circle around the pimple. Blend the edges out with a Q-tip, and dab a tiny bit more concealer on top. Blot very lightly with a tissue.

ASHY SKIN

If you are dark-skinned and prone to an ashy complexion, a few strokes of apricot powder on the face will warm the skin up fast. And, of course, moisturize regularly with a mineral-oil-free lotion.

LASHLESS IN LOUISVILLE

Your cat clawed your leg while you were curling your eyelashes, and you've lost a small chunk of lashes. Go to your local day spa or hair salon and have a ministrand of false lashes attached. You can get an attachment of as few as three strands, which just may do the trick until your lashes grow back.

FACIAL FALLOUT

If your skin looks blotchy and irritated after a facial, apply compresses dipped in chilled chamomile or green tea (or apply the tea bags to your skin). Or, use a product with anti-inflammatory ingredients like green tea, aloe vera, licorice extract, or hydrocortisone to the skin. And next time, schedule a facial a couple of days *before* a big event.

PRODUCTS: Clinique Exceptionally Soothing Cream for Upset Skin ▪ Therapy Systems Emergency Treatment Cream ▪ T. LeClerc Moisture Soothe Serum ▪ Eucerin Redness Relief Daily Perfecting Lotion ▪ Elizabeth Arden Sensitive Skin Calming Moisture Lotion.

WASHED OUT AND WAN

Try Hollywood diva Joan Crawford's remedy for waking up on the set at 6 A.M. Close the drain in the bathroom sink, fill the basin half full with cold water, and add a few drops of lavender oil. With eyes closed, splash handfuls onto your face. Pat your face dry and apply a highlighting lotion.

PRODUCTS: Benefit Cosmetics Hollywood Glo ▪ Revlon Face Illuminator Lotion.

DRY LIPS

Soften dry lips by applying a dab of honey mixed with a bit of sugar. Massage your index finger back and forth across your lips. Wipe or lick off. Yum!

CLUMPY PUMP

Cover the pump on your lotion with foil to prevent clogs and clumps.

What can I do about my shiny face every day about 4 P.M.?

Perk up your face with a spritz of rose water, then lightly blot with a tissue. It will soak up the excess oil, refresh your skin, and help you feel refreshed, too. Or, try a mattifying lotion, especially on the T-zone.

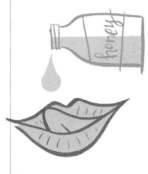

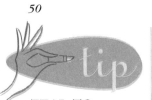

ZEAL TO CONCEAL

Always choose a concealer that's one to two shades lighter than your skin. If you plan to use concealer to camouflage skin problems, look for a dual-pan concealer that contains one light and one darker shade. If you're blending, apply the darker shade to the skin first and blend the lighter shade on top.

PAW PRINTS

You've slept with your makeup on, and now you look like you have two black eyes. What's worse, there's no eye-makeup remover in sight. Head for the kitchen, and put some vegetable oil or butter on a cotton pad or tissue. Gently pat around your eyes. Added bonus: It moisturizes!

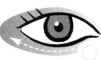

MASCARA MOJO

Touch your fingers or a tissue to your eyes to lift the makeup. Follow it with anything that's emollient—a bit of moisturizer, lip balm, hand cream—to remove the mascara, which will come off much more easily if you take care of it before it dries.

TWEEZER BUMPS

If you get bumps or breakouts after you tweeze, your tweezer may be spreading dirt, oil, and bacteria around. Rinse it with soap and water or wipe it with an antibacterial towelette.

YOU'RE MARKED

The pimple is gone but, alas, not the discoloration and redness that it's left behind. Try a corrective pen like Clinique Acne Solutions Post-Blemish Formula.

THE BODY

What to do when little things go wrong and you're already running late? Your nail chips en route to a party, your manicure messes up, or your makeup cakes onto your suit. A guide to the most common beauty bloopers—from the neck down—and how to get around them!

SCUFFED POLISH

When your toes are on display in sandals, it's no fun to scuff the polish or mess them up with dirt. Carry a portable pack of baby wipes or a travel-size tin of Vaseline, which will remove the dirt in no time.

SNAG HAG

You've torn a nail, and it's snagging all the fine woolens in sight. Clip it, file it, or glue it down with Super Glue.

RATTY NAILS

When your nails look grubby and you need to do something fast, buff them with a soft cloth or massage cuticle oil onto your nails to add shine and a faux "polished" look.

MANI-MESS-CURE

When you apply your nail polish in a hurry, things can get messy. If yours smudges, soak your dry nails in warm water

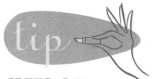

SPEED DRY

The party's starting soon, and your nail polish is still wet. Dip your wet nails in a bowl of ice water (with ice cubes) and keep them there for a minute. Or spray them with Pam.

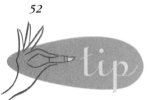

NAIL NURSE

If your nails are stained, mix 2 tablespoons of lemon juice in a cup of warm water. Soak nails for five minutes or longer, as needed. Wipe vigorously with a soft cloth.

for about five minutes, and rub off the smudges with a dry hard-pressed Q-tip or your fingers. Or, dip a Q-tip into a bottle of nail polish remover and dab over the smudge, then touch up the color. Or, try Essie Cuticle Pen, a penlike gizmo that will clean the mess right up.

CRACKING UP

No matter how much gelatin you eat, your nails just crack easily—especially when they're filed. For no-crack nails, gently file yours—in one direction—while the polish is still on. It can help protect them and prevent cracking.

JUST ONE OR TWO CHIPS

It's so annoying when you chip a nail or two and think you need to redo them all. Well, you don't. Put nail polish remover on a Q-tip and smudge it lightly across the chip. Apply a tiny bit of polish to the area. Let it dry for 30 seconds or so. Then, if necessary, brush a thin coat of polish over the entire nail.

NAIL IT

Now that you've—finally!—got your nails looking groomed and polished, what to do when you snag one and it tears? To patch a torn nail, take a tea bag and tear off enough to cover the nail tip and extend it a bit. Apply clear polish over the patch to "glue" it in place. Tuck the end under the nail, and polish.

WAX ON

You've put the wax on your legs, but can't get up the courage to rip it off. Soak in a warm bath for a few minutes; the warmth of the water will loosen the wax. Use a washcloth, gently, to take it off.

SCENTSATIONAL

In France, women know how to apply just enough perfume so that you have to get close to smell it. They also apply it to the hot spots: wrist, throat, that spot behind the knee, and their hair. For great-smelling, long-lasting scented hair, mix a drop of your perfume with your shine serum, and pat it through your hair.

LATER 'GATOR

If your body feels dry, flaky, and truly untouchable before a big date, head for the shower and use a body scrub to exfoliate the dead, flaky skin. If you don't have a scrub, grab a handful of finely ground cornmeal, oatmeal, or even baking soda from the kitchen, put it on a damp washcloth, and gently massage it into your skin. Rinse, pat yourself dry, and moisturize.

MAKEUP ON YOUR DRESS

Rubbing a makeup stain only makes it worse. Instead, put some club soda on a cloth or tissue and press it into the stain. Sprinkle salt on top to soak it up, and brush it off.

Know the spots to apply perfume so your body heat warms and releases the scent.

THE Hair

When life feels overwhelming, it helps to take solace in things that make you feel better, like family, friends, and good hair. These days, the right product—or technique—can fix almost any unhappy hair, and fast!

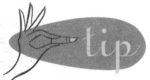

ROOTS REVELATION

When there's no time for a touch-up, dab your mascara wand over your gray roots. Blend it in with an old toothbrush or eyebrow comb. No mascara? You can comb black or brown eye shadow through your roots with a toothbrush. If you're blond, use beige or taupe shadow.

GREASY ROOTS

When you have, literally, one minute, before you need to go, spray your greasy roots with an aerosol hair spray, then give them a ten-second blast with a hot blow-dryer. Or, run blotting papers over your roots—as many as it takes!

HOLD IT

For a long-lasting hold, spritz with a strong-hold hair spray, shake your head upside down, tousle with your fingers, and follow up with a quick blow-dryer blast.

CORKSCREWS UNCORKED

To revive your curly style, spray or pat your hair with a bit of water, which will reactivate the styling products you put on in the morning.

LOCKLUSTER

If your blowout has lost its luster, put back the shine. Slick on a pomade with flecks of shimmer in it.

PRODUCTS: Philip Pelusi Hard Stuff Crystal Gloss ■ Paul Mitchell Gloss Drops ■ Joico K-Pack Protect and Shine Serum.

HALO HIGHLIGHTS

When you think your red or blond hair color needs a lift, dab on a gold or bronze lip gloss (depending on your hair color) and pull through random strands of hair around your face. Comb through with an eyelash comb or old toothbrush.

BROKEN BABY HAIRS

For those little baby hairs that won't stay put and insist on congregating messily along your hairline, put a dab of gel on an old toothbrush and gently brush them back. Or, spray your hair with flexible-hold hair spray and smooth the errant, staticky hairs back with a clean makeup brush.

THE TEXTURIZER

When there are no hair products handy and you want to add a bit of texture to flat, straight hair, take your body lotion—not cream, it's too greasy—and scrunch a quarter-size dab through your hair starting midway down the shaft. Don't start at the roots or your hair will look greasy.

PRODUCT PILE UP

Spray your roots with an aerosol hair spray to absorb excess product.

BOLD AS BRASS

If your highlights are too harsh, shampoo with Dawn liquid dish soap until you can get back to the salon for a redo.

What do I do if I've told the hairstylist what I want, but she does her own thing, and I hate it?

Tell her immediately. Be nice, but explain what you don't like—maybe she can fix it. If not, ask to speak to the manager. Maybe a different stylist can take over. If no one is free, say that you want to come back the next day to see someone else.

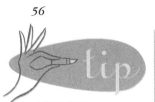

ANIMAL, VEGETABLE . . . MINERAL!

Does your hair always look softer and shinier when you wash it away from home? Hard water can cause mineral buildup on the hair that results in coarse, stiff, dull-looking hair. Wash your hair with a clarifying shampoo to remove mineral deposits.

HELMET HAIR

If you kept your finger on the hair spray trigger for a bit too long and ended up with too much, let it dry, spray your hair with a little water, and tousle.

SLEEP TIGHT

To keep your curly style from frizzing or flattening while you are sleeping, wrap a silk or satin scarf lightly over your head to hold the curl. Finger-fluff it in the morning.

STYLE SOFTENER

When it comes to styling products, always start with less, and add more as you need it. But if you put on too much hair cream, and it looks greasy, spray your hair with a little water, blot with a towel, and style with your fingers.

NO MORE TANGLES?

While you're in the shower, comb through your hair with the conditioner on it. When you get out, your tangles will be gone.

BRIGHT LIGHTS, BAD COLOR

Just like a pair of jeans, your highlights will soften after a few washings. But if they're way too strong and you need to tone them down *now,* wash your hair once or twice with a color-enhancing shampoo in a shade that blends with your natural hair color.

COARSE STRANDS

Turn straw into silk with one of these rich, conditioning hair masks. Then, rinse hair with cold water.

PRODUCTS: Paul Mitchell Instant Moisture Daily Treatment ■ L'Oréal Vive Smooth-Intense Masque.

MUDDY HAIR COLOR

Ever colored your hair at home and ended up with a darker shade than you wanted? The shade pictured on the box is usually one to two shades lighter than the one that shows up on your hair. It's best to have a professional repair the damage. But try this first: Shampoo your hair twice in a row with a clarifying shampoo; it should rinse out some of the color.

OTTER HEAD

If you wash your hair at night and regularly wake up with flat hair, try switching your schedule; wash and condition in the morning instead.

THE BRUSH-OFF

If your round brush gets entangled in your hair, give the brush a couple of blasts of cold air from the blow-dryer, then gently untangle your hair strand by strand. Continue to direct cold blasts downward from the blow-dryer toward the hair on your brush as you untangle. The cold will cause the cuticle to lie flat, which will make it easier to extricate your hair from the brush.

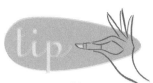

FAKE OUT YOUR HAIR

When there's no time to wash your hair, try this shortcut. Spray leave-in conditioner on the ends and around the face (to take down flyaways and frizz). Blast with a blow-dryer for a minute or two. Instant softness and shine!

CALL IT SPLITS

You need to get your split ends cut, but in the meantime, pull a smoothing serum through the ends of your hair, and blast them with a cold shot from your blow-dryer to seal them.

CANOPY BANGS

Put a dime-size dab of hair balm or pomade in your palm to warm it up, then take sections of your bangs and pull the product through. Or, massage the product through bangs, and tie a scarf, tightly, around your head for a few minutes.

PRODUCTS: Aveda Control Paste ■ Redken Water Wax.

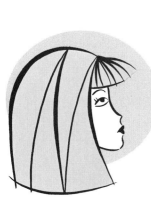

In humid weather, bangs can spiral out of control.

DRY, FRIZZY ENDS

Pull a bit of leave-in conditioner through the ends of your hair.

SQUEAKY CLEAN

If your hair is consistently heavy and dull, maybe you don't rinse it well enough. Spend some extra time under your shower nozzle. For really shiny hair, rinse it in cool water for about 90 seconds—until your hair squeaks—before you condition.

FRIGHT NIGHT

You work up a sweat as you walk to work on a humid day, and, when you get there, your hair looks like Madeline Kahn's in *Young Frankenstein*. Spritz your palms a

fast guide for brides

Special occasions, like weddings, require planning ahead, but no matter how much time you put into your preparation, real life inevitably intrudes, resulting in last-minute glitches that need fast fixes.

PHOTO FINISH

To have your makeup last and look great in your wedding photos:

1 Choose a light-reflecting foundation, or mix your foundation with a highlighter before you apply.

PRODUCTS: Clinique Zero Base ■ L'Oréal Translucide Lasting Luminous Makeup ■ Clarins True Radiance Foundation.

2 Don't forget your powder compact, for shine-free photos.

3 Make sure your mascara is waterproof, for obvious reasons. Since waterproof mascara is apt to be gunky, comb through your lashes with an old toothbrush.

4 Lipstick with brown tones can look really flat in photos. Not a good choice.

5 Stick with cream blush to warm up your skin. It lasts longer—and you'll have lots of other things on your mind besides touch-ups.

6 Keep your chin up, it's the most flattering angle.

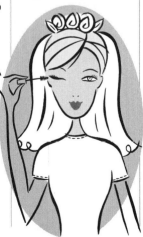

PLAN-AHEAD TIPS:

1 If you plan to wear flowers in your hair, apply hairspray *before* you put the flowers in, or else the spray will wilt the flowers.

2 When you do a test run for your bridal makeup, wear a white T-shirt to make sure the palette you've chosen will flatter you in your wedding gown.

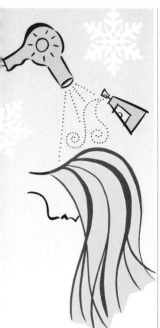

couple of times with a nonaerosol hair spray. Pat your hands through your hair.

FLAT AS A PANCAKE

If your hair has fallen like a soufflé, turn your head upside down, spray volumizer into the roots, and shoot it with a blast or two of cool air for instant body. Toss back your head, shake your hair and go.

PRODUCTS: Aveda Confixer Volumizer Spray Gel ▪ Phyto Phytovolume Actif Volumizer Spray.

STYLE SHORTCUT

When you don't have time to finish styling, leave the back of your hair and focus on the front—your hairline and the top of your head. The rest will fall into place on its own.

The cool setting on a blow-dryer does the least damage to your hair.

MAKING WAVES

If you want loose waves but don't have time for styling, simply pull your damp hair into a low ponytail and braid it in a loose braid down to the end or twist your hair into a bun before bed. Let it dry naturally.

PART II:

hormonal
hangups

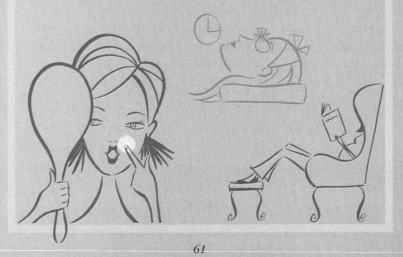

CHAPTER FOUR

Tweens and Teens (Puberty)

UBERTY IS THE RITE OF PASSAGE FROM CHILDHOOD to adulthood. It can be a stressful time, because your hormones are going wild and causing profound changes in your body, your behavior, and your moods. The word *hormone* comes from the ancient Greek *hormao*, which means "to arouse to activity." In other words, hormones are the body's little agitators.

During puberty, you sweat more, your skin breaks out, and your hair is greasy. Your body is changing, your moods are swinging, your social life is a roller coaster, *and* you've got a mountain of homework! As if that's not enough, suddenly you care more than ever about looking good. A pimple is nothing short of catastrophic. Shaving bumps are *so* embarrassing. Frizzy hair is not acceptable, period. Oh, and speaking of your period, let's not forget about bloat, oily skin, B.O., and the insecurity that goes along with not knowing how to deal with any of it.

But before we even begin to talk about fast fixes on the outside, I want to make an important point. Beauty—for both girls and boys—begins below the surface. Beauty begins in the brain. If you can focus on feeling better about yourself (rather than picking yourself apart) you'll look better, too.

ACNE

D id you know that more than 70 percent of all teenagers develop acne? That may not make you feel better as you struggle to deal with breakouts, but it's good to know that acne is normal, and that it will pass. Acne hits boys harder because most teenage acne is caused when hyperactive oil glands, stimulated by the male hormone androgen, mix with dead skin cells to clog pores. Androgen production is highest during the teen years, and, obviously, guys produce more androgen. Of course, many girls break out on a regular basis each month before their period. But both sexes will find that acne is

A.M.

1. Cleanse: Alternate a liquid cleanser (for oily skin) with cleansing pads.

2. Moisturize: With an oil-free moisturizer to keep skin from overdrying.

3. Medicate: Girls: Apply medicated concealer to blemishes; guys: apply a clear acne medication to blemishes.

P.M.

1. Cleanse

2. Exfoliate: Use a facial scrub to remove pore-clogging detritus that leads to blackheads and pimples. Don't rub! Gently press the scrub into your skin.

3. Medicate: Apply spot medication to blemishes.

gender neutral when it comes to bad timing, which must be why zits always seem to pop up the day before a big date or a party. Here's how to beat back the zits.

ON-THE-SPOT MEDICATIONS

There are many antiacne medications for severe acne, and some, like the retinoids (vitamin A derivatives)—Differin, Tazorac, Retin-A—are available by prescription only. If your acne is severe, visit a dermatologist. But for normal breakouts, look for a drying lotion with up to 2 percent salicylic acid like Bye-Bye Blemish Drying Lotion or Herbalogic. For a more natural option, look for products with tea tree oil or parsley.

PRODUCTS: Burt's Bee's Herbal Blemish Stick ■ Osea Essential Corrective Complex ■ Desert Essence Blemish Touch Stick ■ Ole Henriksen Roll-On Blemish Attack ■ Swabplus Advanced Acne Care Swabs.

NIP IT IN THE BUD

When you feel a pimple coming, wrap an ice cube in a thin cloth or paper towel and hold it to the area, off and on, for 15 minutes. Or, leave a dab of clay face mask on it for 30 minutes—or overnight.

BLACKHEAD BUSTERS

Don't pick or you can scar! A dermatologist or facialist can remove blackheads, or you can try these remedies. Spread Elmer's Glue on blackheads, let it dry, and peel it off. Blackheads peel off too, if they're not too deep. (See page 256 for a blackhead-loosening steam 'n scrub.)

PRODUCT: Biore Deep Cleaning Pore Strips.

SUPER-SIZED PORES

Apply plain, chilled yogurt to your face for ten minutes, then rinse with cool water. It feels really refreshing, absorbs excess oil and bacteria, and helps make your pores look smaller.

PRODUCTS: Neutrogena Pore Refining Lotion ■ Shiseido Pureness Anti-Shine Refreshing Lotion.

DARK SPOTS

After a blemish goes away, the dark spot may not. Try Clinique Acne Solutions Post-Blemish Formula or Miracle II Neutralizing Gel, and it will.

UNDERCOVER

To cover random pimples, look for a medicated concealer (with salicylic acid) that will cover the blemish and help eradicate it at the same time.

PRODUCTS: Clinique Acne Solutions Concealing Cream ■ Neutrogena SkinClearing Oil-Free Concealer ■ Benefit Cosmetics Galactic Shield.

MAKEUP BREAKOUTS

If it seems that your skin breaks out after you wear a certain makeup—especially foundation—some of the ingredients may be clogging your pores. Look for makeup that

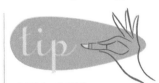

OUT, OUT, DAMN SPOT!

Apply a dab of calamine lotion or Milk of Magnesia to the blemish at bedtime, and it will be gone by morning. Or, dab some honey on your pimple, cover it with a Band-Aid, and go to bed. Honey kills bacteria and hastens the healing process.

KITCHEN SINK SPOT TREATMENTS

■ Cut a clove of garlic in half and, no kidding, dab on your pimple once or twice a day. Garlic kills bacteria and also kills pimples. Don't apply to open pimples.

■ Mix a teaspoon of red wine vinegar into a cup of water, and dab on spot blemishes, but not on open pimples.

■ Place a thin slice of potato on the pimple at bedtime, secure it with a Band-Aid, and remove it in the morning.

is labeled oil-free or noncomedogenic instead.

IT'S TIGHT AND WHITE

Apply Neosporin (or any over-the-counter antibiotic ointment) to a tight, angry whitehead or pimple before you go to bed.

OVERNIGHT AND OUT OF SIGHT

Apply a peel-away patch before you go to bed, and the salicylic acid in it will reduce the size of the blemish by the morning.

PRODUCTS: Biore Blemish Bomb ■ Phisoderm Blemish Patch.

THE T-ZONE

To get rid of shine—especially around the T-Zone—use a mattifier or oil-blotting product that can absorb excess oil and keep your skin shine-free all day (see page 128).

HAIRLINE PIMPLES

Acne on the forehead can be caused by hair conditioners or styling products, which can clog pores. Don't let these products get on your skin. If you must, wear a headband on the area from your hairline to your forehead when you're styling your hair. Baseball caps can also trap dirt and sweat and cause breakouts. Make sure that you keep yours clean.

PIECE OF MAGIC

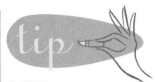

An alum block is a little piece of magic with many uses. Dampen it and lightly rub it over a whitehead, and its salt deposits will clear up the whitehead overnight. Rub a pimple with an alum block twice a day.

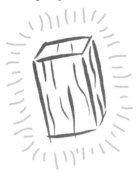

Alum also works as a deodorant and stops small cuts from bleeding. Where to find it? www.eshave.com, health-food stores, and the drugstore, where it may be called "styptic" or styptic pencil.

MINI BREAKOUT

For a minibreakout, apply diaper rash cream (with zinc oxide) to the area before you go to bed, and rinse it off in the morning.

Face it

Face it: Life feels a little bit random at the moment, and so does your skin. You sweat more, your oil glands are getting worked up, your face looks really shiny, and it's freaking you out. Even if you don't have blackheads or pimples, your skin just doesn't look as good as it once did, but with a few simple tricks and changes in your routine, things will get back to normal.

MISS SENSITIVE

If your skin flushes easily or reacts badly (you get a rash, redness, or breakout) when you try different skincare products, you may have sensitive skin (see page 234). Avoid lotions that are heavily fragranced or contain essential oils (these are natural, but

fast funky face masks

Here are some fast, foodie-based blemish-busting face masks. If you prefer *not* to make it yourself, look for commercial products with kaolin (clay), tea tree oil, sulfur, camphor, lycopene (from tomatoes), or willow bark (a source for salicylic acid) in their ingredient lists.

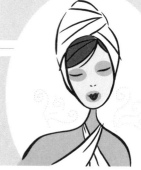

■ Mash the pulp of a small piece of **watermelon**. Apply it to your entire face and leave on till it tightens and the juice dries (about ten minutes). Wash with warm water, then rinse with cool water.

■ Cut a **tomato** in half. Massage it on your face. Let it dry, then rinse. Don't apply to open pimples, as it may sting.

■ Grate an **apple** and mix it with 2 teaspoons of **honey**. Apply to a breakout area and leave on for 15 minutes. Rinse with warm, then cool water.

■ Soak a small piece of **bread** in **milk**. Lie down, place it on the pimple, and leave it for 20 minutes.

■ Mix a squirt of **mint toothpaste** (not gel) in your palm with a few drops of warm water. Dab on blemishes, and leave on for five minutes. Rinse with cool water.

some can irritate sensitive skin). Other irritants include lanolin, mint menthol, camphor, enzymes, and alpha hydroxy acid.

MUSTACHE FUZZ

One of the more embarrassing teen developments can be the growth of facial hair, which may darken and hint at a mustache. No problem if you're a guy, but if you're a girl, it's not so cool. When you get older, you can wax your upper lip, if you like, or consider electrolysis or laser treatments. But for now, a quick way to camouflage lip hair is to bleach it. Get a box of Jolene Cream Bleach from the drugstore, and follow directions. Don't leave it on too long; it can burn your skin!

TOO YOUNG TO TWEEZE

If your brows are wild, but you're too young to start tweezing, try a clear brow gel (or Vaseline) to tame them. Brow gels look just like mascara—they even come with a wand applicator—but the goop is clear. Wipe the wand around the edge of the tube and stroke it on your brows in an upward direction. If it looks too stiff after it dries, brush your brows with an old toothbrush.

METAL MOUTH

If you're self-conscious about your braces, move the focus away from your mouth and onto your eyes. Experiment with eye shadow, curl your lashes, and apply a bit of mascara.

After I go to the beach, I get lots of freckles. My mom has tons. How can I prevent them?

The best way to minimize freckles is to use a broad-spectrum sunscreen with SPF 15, with titanium dioxide or zinc oxide listed as an active ingredient. Or, grow to love them—they're really cute (see page 93)!

When I stay up late studying, I have dark circles under my eyes the next day. How can I cover them up?

To cover dark circles, pat a cream concealer under your eyes. (The concealer needs to be one or two shades lighter than your skin because your circles are darker than your skin.) Pat the concealer on with your fourth finger and blend it well. Brush a bit of powder on top.

SHAMPOO TIP FOR SENSITIVE SKIN

Try to hold your head back when you rinse out your shampoo. Shampoo contains ingredients that are generally harsher than skincare ingredients, and they can irritate your face——especially if your skin is sensitive.

SORE-LIP SOOTHER

Take a wet tea bag (make sure to use green or black tea, not an herbal variety) and hold it against your irritated lips for a couple of minutes. The tannic acid in the tea soothes the skin and helps it heal fast.

BAD BREATH

Most of the bacteria that cause bad breath live on the tongue. If you want to sweeten your breath, brush your tongue. Or, if you're not near your toothbrush, eat an apple. Biting into the crisp, fibrous flesh cleans the teeth, while the pectin in the apple neutralizes the bad odor.

LIP LOSS

Color your lips in with a pencil, and top with lip balm to make color last.

SWOLLEN EYELIDS

If your eyelids swell after you've started using your new eyelash curler, you might be allergic to the nickel plating that's commonly used on the edge. Stop using it for a couple of days and see if the swelling goes down. Or, visit a dermatologist.

YOU'RE BLUSHING

When the blood vessels in your face dilate, you blush. To stop the embarrassing flush, hold a washcloth dipped in cool water against your face. Or, if you're feeling stressed or anxious, try a classic yoga technique—breathe in through the nose and out through the mouth—to calm your anxiety. Hot, spicy food and alcohol can also make your skin flush.

SLIPPERY LIP GLOSS

When your lip gloss won't stay on your lips (this happens with certain drugstore brands), smooth an ice cube over your lips on top of the gloss.

PALE FACE

No color on your cheeks and no blush in the house? Do what your grandma did: Rub a dab of lipstick on your cheeks.

PAINLESS PLUCKING

The first couple of times you tweeze your brows can hurt, and the area can be sensitive. If your eyes are tearing from the pain of plucking (especially if you're an eyebrow virgin), apply a warm compress for a few seconds, then tweeze. Repeat until finished. Or, massage a bit of Anbesol on the area to numb it before you tweeze. When you're done, apply ice until the skin calms down.

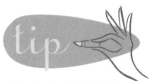

SOFT SQUEEZE

Choose tweezers with flexible plastic tips instead of metal. Plastic tips are sharp enough to grip the hair, but not as sharp as metal, and less likely to rough up the skin.

Bad Hair Days

All of a sudden, your hair has gone from glossy to greasy. And, if you've colored it, it may feel as dry as straw. No matter how many gels, mousses, creams, or conditioners you buy, no matter how much time you spend in the bathroom with your blow-dryer, your hair still doesn't look like you want it to look. That's because your body is changing, and so is your hair.

HANDMADE HEADBAND

To keep your hair off your face when you're doing your makeup, cut a strip across the leg of your holey black pantyhose and use it as a stretch headband. It's even cute enough to wear outdoors.

BABY-FINE BLUES

To give your baby-fine hair more body, reverse the natural order: condition first, and then shampoo.

PRODUCTS: Phyto Phytovolume Maximizing Volume Shampoo ■ Pantene Pro-V Sheer Volume Conditioner ■ Neutrogena Clean Volume Shampoo.

OILY ROOTS

Mix equal amounts of water and alcohol-free toner in a spray bottle, shake it to blend, and spritz on your roots. Then blow-dry.

OILY HAIR

Tea tree oil (or rosemary) shampoo will help absorb excess oil. Or, mix a tiny drop of tea tree oil—a great natural astringent—into a palmful of your usual shampoo, then wash.

PRODUCTS: Paul Mitchell Tea Tree Hair and Body Moisturizer ■ Avalon Organics Botanicals Volumizing Rosemary Shampoo.

GREASY ROOTS

Massage a half-teaspoon of baby powder or corn starch into your roots, turn your head upside down, and fluff at the roots. (These will blend in better if your hair is blond. If your hair is brown, use a bit of bronzing powder instead.)

OIL-PROOF YOUR HAIR

Use a gentle, everyday shampoo formulated for oily hair. Rather than massage your scalp, press it with the flat part of your fingers. Ditto for combing and brushing—don't rub the scalp too vigorously, or you'll stimulate the glands to produce more oil.

PRODUCTS: Citrus shampoos with orange or lemon ■ Kerastase Bain Antigras ■ Nivea Anti-Oily Shampoo ■ John Masters Organics Lemongrass Oily Hair Shampoo.

SUDDENLY GREASY?

If you've recently started using a medicated shampoo for dandruff or greasiness—stop. These can overdry the scalp long enough for it to start oversecreting oil again, making your hair even greasier. After shampooing, rinse with a cup of peppermint tea, which has steeped until strong and cooled. Leave it in, do not rinse out. Style hair as usual.

SMELLY HAIR

To get rid of gross smells that have attached themselves to your hair (like stinky food or cigarette smoke), wipe a fabric softener sheet like Bounce through your hair.

I heard that it's bad to share your makeup with friends. Is that true?

Don't ever share eye makeup because you risk getting an eye infection. Sharing lipstick can lead to cold sores and infections, too. Even though cosmetics contain preservatives that should kill bacteria, it's not a good idea.

My hair is bleaching along my hairline and I don't know why.

If you are using a benzoyl peroxide antiacne product on your face, don't let it slip up onto your hair! Benzoyl peroxide can bleach hair along with your clothes and towels. Warning: Don't use benzoyl peroxide and tretinoin (a vitamin A derivative) at the same time. It can leave your skin irritated and overly sensitive to the sun.

It will absorb the odor and leave your hair stink-free.

TANGLED UP

If your hair tends to tangle, condition it in the shower. Let the conditioner soak in for a minute while you wash your body. Then, comb through your hair—while still in the shower—with a wide-toothed comb. Rinse.

FRIGHT-NIGHT HAIR

If your hair is standing on end, take a dab of moisturizing lotion or lip balm in your palms and pat it through the ends of your hair. Or, run a sheet of fabric softener through staticky hair. Or, spray Static Guard on your hairbrush or inside your hat.

STATICKY STUFF

Blot your hair dry with a towel after you shampoo and before you condition. Your hair will absorb the conditioner better, which will protect it from static.

FLYAWAYS

Spray your hair with a flexible hold or nonaerosol pump hair spray, and run a shaving brush or natural-bristle makeup brush over your hair to smooth. Or, try a wax-based hair spray. These work like pomade, but because they spray on, they are distributed lightly and don't weigh the hair down.

PRODUCTS: Paul Mitchell Spray Wax ■ TIGI Headbanger.

STIFF BRUSH

Overbrushing leads to staticky hair, and a cheap new brush with really stiff bristles can rough up your hair and really create static. Heat the bristles with your blow-dryer to soften them, then brush.

TOO MUCH GEL?

If you've put on too much gel and have no time to wash it out, run a towel over your hair a couple of times.

FA FRIZZLE

If your curly hair is frizz-prone, use a moisturizing shampoo and conditioner for dry hair. To minimize frizz when styling, run a styling cream through damp hair.

PRODUCTS: Pantene Pro-V Frizz Control Crème ▪ Bumble and bumble Curl Conscious ▪ Kiehls Creme with Silk Groom ▪ Lavett & Chin Shea Butter Hair Crème ▪ L'Oréal Anti-Frizz Cream ▪ Garnier Fructis Sleek & Shine Weightless Anti-Frizz Serum.

THE OPPOSITE OF PERM

If your hair is thin and stick-straight, and you want to make it look fuller, you can (1) cut it in layers, which will add texture and dimension to flat hair, and (2) apply volumizer to your roots and ends, and focus on those areas when you blow your hair dry.

THE BIG AND BRASSY

To protect highlights, spray on a leave-in conditioner when in the sun. Look for silicone ingredients ending in "-one."

SPLIT ENDS

Split ends result from roughing up your hair with your brush, comb, or other styling tools. If you've got 'em:

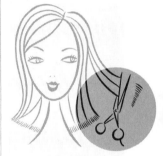

1. Cut 'em off.

2. "Piece" your ends together temporarily with hair wax or pomade.

3. Apply a light silicone styling product and direct the blow-dryer on your ends for a sec.

4. Warm a bit of olive oil, squeeze it into your ends, and give them a quick blast with your dryer.

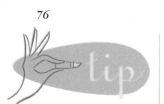

GO WITH THE BLOW

Keep the blow-dryer moving as you go. Too much hot air in one place can really fry your hair.

WHEN YOUR CURLS ARE LOSING IT

Spray a curl activator on your hair to rejuvenate your curls.

PRODUCTS: L'Oréal Pumping Curls ▪ Pantene Pro-V Curl Revive Frizz Control Treatment ▪ Ouidad Botanical Boost.

HOT HEAD

If you blow-dry or flat-iron your hair straight on a regular basis—stop. At least give your hair the weekend off from heat styling. Use the low setting on your blow-dryer, instead of high, and spray with a heat protection product before you style it.

PRODUCTS: Paul Mitchell Heat Seal ▪ Neutrogena HeatSafe.

FRIED HAIR

Don't blow-dry your hair when it's sopping wet. Blot your hair dry with a towel first; you'll cut down on your blow-drying time, and you'll have healthier hair.

ROUGH HAIR

Massage your hair with olive oil, wrap it in Saran Wrap or cover it with a shower cap, give it a quick blast with the blow-dryer to seal moisture into the hair cuticle, leave it on for about 20 minutes, then shampoo and condition your hair.

GLOOPY GOOP

Always apply hairstyling products to your hands first, never directly on your hair.

color-treated hair

Your hair is made up of approximately 98 percent protein. When it's overprocessed by chemical treatments, the proteins break down, the hair loses water, and it becomes dry and brittle. For healthier hair color:

1 Look for semi-permanent rather than permanent hair color—these use fewer harsh chemicals, which can rough up your hair.

2 Look for ammonia-free (or low-ammonia), low-PPD dyes. Ammonia and PPD (p-phenylenediamene) help color stick to the hair shaft, but they can be irritating to the skin and dry out the hair, so use as little as possible.

3 Try vegetable-based color or henna. Veggie-based color doesn't last as long as conventional color, and it isn't easy to get a subtle look with henna, but they won't damage your hair. Veggie-based hair color: Herbatint, Naturtint, Aveda Color Current Energized Gel Color, Light Mountain Natural Henna Hair Color.

4 If your hair is damaged, wash with shampoo for color-treated hair, use a moisturizing conditioner, and give yourself a deep-conditioning treatment once a week to help put moisture back into your hair.

PRODUCTS FOR COLOR-TREATED HAIR:

- John Masters Organics Evening Primrose Shampoo for Dry Hair
- Pureology Purify Shampoo and Conditioner
- L'oreal Vive Hi-Light Boosting Shampoo
- Aveda Color Conserve Shampoo
- Aveda Color Conserve Conditioner
- Aura Cacia Color Extending Shampoo
- Paul Mitchell Color Protect Reconstructive Treatment
- Angela Cosmai Daily Shampoo and Conditioner
- Clairol Herbal Essence Replenishing Shampoo
- Clairol Herbal Essence Replenishing Conditioner

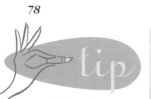

PRODUCT OVERLOAD

Experimenting with lots of hairstyling products can sometimes lead to dull-looking hair. Use a clarifying shampoo once a week—or rinse your hair with a teaspoon of vinegar diluted in a cup of water—and hey, lighten up on the gels, mousses, and hair sprays.

Then, use your hands to apply the product and a comb to distribute it evenly from roots to ends.

BAD BANGS

The secret to great-looking bangs is to have them trimmed every six weeks. (Most stylists will do this for free as long as you go to them for your haircut.) Take two minutes in the morning, dampen your bangs, take a round fat brush, roll the brush under, and blow them until dry.

SCALP BREAKOUTS

Don't apply shampoo or conditioner directly to your head. First, apply shampoo to your hands, massage it through your hair, then massage it into your scalp with the flats of your fingers. Keep conditioner off the scalp and on the hair from midpoint to ends.

THICK TO THIN

The most common cause of thinning hair in teens is overprocessing. If you color, straighten, or perm your hair, stop. Give your hair a break. While you're on your style sabbatical, use Pantene Full and Thick Shampoo and Conditioner to make hair look thicker. Take a multiple vitamin and if your hair doesn't grow back, see a dermatologist.

BODY WOES

In every culture—even in many different species!—puberty is celebrated as a rite of passage, but it feels like a bubbling, roiling, biological stew. It may be hard to celebrate certain unwelcome body changes like BO, hairy legs, cramps, butt bumps, and bacne. With these easy tips, you'll not only get used to it, you'll get it all back under control.

NAIL BITES

It's a lot easier—and more tempting—to bite your nails when the skin surrounding them is dry. Use a hand cream, cuticle oil, or vegetable oil to moisturize your cuticles. When your hands are moisturized, you will be less tempted to damage your digits.

TIGHT SKIN ACROSS YOUR BREASTS

You're growing and your skin is stretching. Apply a light body lotion to your buds to make them feel better. Don't worry if one bud looks bigger than the other— it will even out. But in the meantime, if it bothers you, buy a bra with removable pads so that you can balance things out a bit.

UNDERARM STUBBLE

Your underarm hair grows in several different directions. To shave it all off, shave in different directions—upward, downward, then sideways to get every last bit of stubble.

My soap leaves a gross film on my skin. What can I do?

It sounds like your household has hard water whose minerals can cause soap to leave a scum on your skin. It can also make skin feel dry and itchy. Switch to a "soapless" soap or shower gel. Or, ask your parents to switch to soft water.

TEEN FUZZ-BUSTERS

These are the quickest routes to smooth and stubble-free hair removal.

Depilatory cream: Look for a product with soothing chamomile or aloe to counter irritation.

Waxing: Salons often use hot wax, but it takes a lot of courage to use it on yourself. Cold wax strips are the best bet (least mess and discomfort) for at-home waxers.

Shaving: For the smoothest shave, let shaving cream or gel sit on your skin for a minute or two before shaving.

Mitts: Abrasive mitts (a manual depilatory) massage legs free of hair and razor stubble.

BUTT BUMPS

The skin on your behind is twice as thick as the skin on your face. If you have hard bumps back there, it may be keratosis pilaris (K.P.) which looks like acne without the whiteheads. It comes from chafing due to tight clothing, less-than-stellar hygiene, or no fault of your own. Exfoliate with a natural-bristle brush or body scrub in the shower, and use a body lotion with glycolic acid on the area.

BUTT BREAKOUTS

These can be triggered by genetics or sweat that traps bacteria and leads to clogged pores. Apply spot medication to the pimples, and apply a blemish-busting clay face mask (that's right, *face* mask!) with kaolin or bentonite in the ingredients list.

PRODUCTS: Origins Get Down ■ Alba Botanica Deep Sea Facial Mask ■ Beauty Without Cruelty Facial Mask, Purifying.

RAZOR BURNS

Shave with a thin coat of Vaseline instead of shaving cream to prevent irritation. In a pinch, use hair conditioner. If your armpits get irritated when you apply deodorant after shaving, wait at least 15 minutes to apply. If you're prone to razor burn, try Rash Decision by Oloff Beauty.

BLAME THE BLADE

Old, overused blades can become a breeding ground for bacteria. Make

TATTOO YOU

Tattoo artists inject color into your skin with a needle attached to a motor that holds up to 14 needles with pigments. Some tattoos are applied by hand. Depending on the tattoo, the process takes anywhere from 15 minutes to several months to complete.

According to the FDA (Food and Drug Administration), these are potential problems that can arise when you get a tattoo.

1. Infection. Needles that aren't sterile can transmit infectious diseases like hepatitis or even HIV.

2. Allergic reactions. Reactions to the colors used in tattoos are rare, but they do happen.

3. Granulomas. Raised nodules that can form around foreign substances in the body, such as tattoo pigments.

4. Keloids. These are scars that can form from a tattoo or from removal of a tattoo.

5. Complications with removal. Getting rid of a tattoo takes several treatments, and there is a risk of scarring.

Before you get a tattoo, think about how hard it will be to remove if you change your mind. Lasers are the most popular method of removal—which can be pricey and painful—along with surgery or dermabrasion.

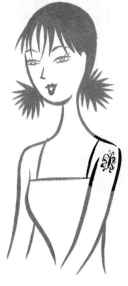

sure to rinse your blade after every use, and don't stretch your blades any longer than a couple of shaves.

HAIR-LESS

Your leg hair is becoming coarse and dark, and you want to shave less often. Try a hair regrowth inhibitor cream. These are moisturizers with soy protein (or an enzyme called papain). After three or four weeks, the hair grows in softer and lighter.

PRODUCT: Jergens Naturally Smooth Shave Minimizing Moisturizer.

TATTOOS YOU LOSE

To cover up your body art, use a heavy cream foundation or concealer. You'll need two shades: one that's a couple of shades lighter than your skin—light enough to apply directly to the tattoo as a concealer—and one darker shade that matches your skin tone. Apply with a brush, and keep the makeup directly on the tattoo. Top with powder, and buff with a powder brush.

PRODUCTS: Dermablend Coverage Cosmetics Leg and Body Cover Creme ■ M·A·C Face and Body Foundation.

HAIR LINES

If you want to wear a bikini but you're embarrassed by a line of hair that runs from your navel to your nether regions, you

B.O. BITES

During puberty, hormones activate the sweat glands under your arms and cause you to sweat more, smell worse, and stain your clothes. The sweat mixes with bacteria to cause body odor. It's totally normal, but most teens aren't exactly comfortable with it. Here are some things to know:

■ Deodorant masks body odor with other, perfumey smells, but doesn't stop wetness. Antiperspirant causes cells lining your sweat ducts to swell and close, which prevents the release of sweat and reduces wetness.

Most drugstore brands are a combination of both.

■ Natural deodorant contains odor-breaking plant extracts like coriander, lavender, sage, and witch hazel as active ingredients.

PRODUCTS: Dr. Hauschka Skin Care Deodorant Fresh ■ Weleda Deodorant ■ Tom's of Maine Natural Deodorant.

Tip: You can also use an alum block (see page 67) to absorb odor.

can wax it, bleach it, and eventually remove it entirely with electrolysis or laser treatments.

NO-PAIN GAIN

If it hurts when you wax, take an Advil or Motrin half an hour before you start.

PIERCING PROBLEM

If you just got a piercing and the area looks swollen, itchy, and perhaps oozy with fluid, you may have allergic contact dermatitis, an inflammation reaction caused by contact with a substance that doesn't agree with your skin. It's not uncommon to have an allergy to nickel or other metals in posts used for piercing. Call your doctor for advice.

GROWTH SPURTS

Stretchmarks may appear with a sudden growth spurt. Girls may see thick red lines across their breasts. Sudden weight gain is another common cause of stretch marks. Massage the area twice a day with a rich moisturizer or gel.

PRODUCTS: Sothys Freshening Gel ■ StriVectin SD.

THE TEEN SLUMP

Bad posture is so endemic that most teens aren't even aware of it. Just take a 50-pound backpack loaded with books, and you've got the slump. To look taller and stand up straighter, try this: Imagine that you're holding a tennis ball between your shoulder blades. Now, don't drop it.

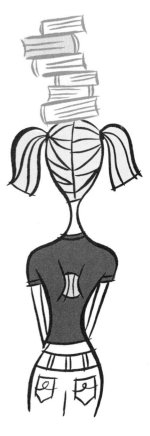

Breathing deeply into your diaphragm makes you automatically stand up straighter.

your period

In the early years of adolescence, when your flow can be inconsistent, your skin may seem to break out always at the least opportune times—prom night, graduation, a big date—you get the picture! As your period becomes more regular, there's a good chance you'll also be able to count on cramps and breakouts on your back and chest—if you don't get them already. And then, of course, there's PMS, along with its attendant backaches, headaches, breast soreness, bloating, moodiness, and fatigue. It's a wild ride until your cycle evens out and you know what to expect each month—and how to make yourself look and feel better.

YOU FEEL BLOATED

Eating ginger, garlic, or papaya is great for reducing bloat. To brew a cup of ginger tea, fill a small saucepan with water, slice in some hunks of ginger, and let it simmer for at least ten minutes.

A HAIRY MOMENT

Don't use a depilatory right before or right after your period—your skin will be more sensitive and may break out.

WAX AND WHINE

The worst time to wax is when you have your period. Wait until the week after your period, when your hormone levels go down. It will be far less painful, and your skin will be less sensitive and less prone to splotches, rashes, or raised bumps that look like chicken skin. The same goes for eyebrow tweezing.

A PLUS-SIZE PORE

Large pores seem to loom larger on your face during your period. Use a clay mask

PMS: THE FOOD PLAN

PMS is thought to be caused by increased levels of progesterone, which lead to cramps, edginess, bloating, breast tenderness, depression, headaches, and constipation—symptoms we've all read about on the back of the Mydol box.

Because progesterone causes water retention—which not only makes you bloat, it can make you edgy—you can relieve symptoms by eating more diuretic (salt- and water-flushing) foods like cucumber, asparagus, parsley, celery, and leafy green vegetables. Drink a lot of water. Avoid foods like avocado, chocolate, soy sauce, and aged cheese, as they are high in tyramine, a substance that raises blood pressure. To ease constipation, increase your fiber intake and eat more whole grains, raw fruits, and raw vegetables. Vitamin B6 (a diuretic and enzyme in endorphin production) can help with mood swings and edginess; vitamin E and calcium supplements also may make you feel better, though no one really knows why. Too much caffeine (more than two cups of coffee per day) will make you jumpy.

the week of your period—it will tighten the skin and make your pores appear smaller.

PRODUCTS: Neutrogena Pore Refining Mask ▪ Avon Pore-Minimizing Mask ▪ Kiss My Face Pore Shrink Deep Cleansing Mask ▪ Clinique Pore Minimizer Refining Lotion.

CRAMPS

Red raspberry leaf, lemon balm, and chamomile teas relax cramps. Exercise and yoga help, along with calcium and vitamin B6. Lie down with a warm (almost hot) towel covering your pelvic area for about ten minutes. Sprinkle a few drops of lavender essential oil on the towel, which will help your body to relax.

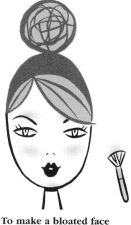

To make a bloated face look less full, brush bronzing powder onto temples, cheekbones, and under your chin.

beauty myths

Some beauty myths, passed down through generations of women, seem to have taken on a life of their own. Here are a few of the most common, with the reasons why they're false. (Ask your mom if she's heard of any of these.)

Someone told me that if I use a ponytail, my hair can break and fall out.

Pulling your hair back really tightly every day can put stress on it, and it can break off. The same is true for tight braids and twists, but you shouldn't have a problem if you wear those styles only occasionally. Don't pull your hair back tightly all of the time, and don't use uncoated elastics or elastics with metal clasps, which can cause breakage.

French fries, chocolate, pizza, chips, and other foods make your skin break out.

Though you don't want to overload on any of these because they are full of sugar, salt, or fat, no food has been scientifically proven to cause breakouts. If your face always breaks out when you eat pizza or chips, well, don't eat them. You may have a food allergy.

Bad hygiene causes pimples.

In fact, many people with pimples tend to wash their skin too hard and too often, which can strip oil from the skin and cause your body to secrete even more oil to compensate—leading to skin that's both dry and pimply! Wash your face with cleanser twice a day—in the morning and at night—and rinse with water more often if you like.

Lots of lather means that my shampoo is working better.

You may like extra foam on your latte, but excess lather from your shampoo does not mean that it's doing a better job. It probably means that the product contains extra foaming agents to make it lather up, but it isn't making your hair cleaner—and it may not be as gentle as a low-lather shampoo.

It's bad to mix different brands of skincare and cosmetics.

This is a marketing ploy that must have been started by a cosmetics exec to encourage loyalty to one brand. You don't feel like you have to wear one brand of clothing from head to toe, do you? In fact, it's good to mix things up. Some companies make some products extremely well, and not others.

Cutting your hair makes it grow faster.

Your hair grows at the roots, not the ends. If your hair is short, you will notice it more when it grows, but that's about it.

Sun exposure clears up acne.

When you tan, your acne may look less obvious, but tanned skin is drier and causes the skin to stimulate more oil, which can cause more pimples. Plus, many acne medications make the skin sensitive to the sun, and the interaction can make you break out or develop a rash.

Shaving your legs makes the hair grow in thicker.

Shaving may make your hair *look* thicker when it grows back, because the razor blunts the ends and your hair becomes more visible. However, you are genetically prewired for each and every hair on your body, and that's all you get—no more, and no less, unless hormonal changes or medication cause it to change.

You can make your pores smaller.

You can make your pores *look* smaller by plumping the surrounding skin with moisturizer or by using certain types of "pore-refining" lotions or makeup. On the other hand, when a pore is clogged with a blackhead, bacteria, or dead skin, it can stretch and appear bigger until it's unclogged. But your pores are not like a door or window that you can open or shut.

Wash your hair twice when you shampoo.

Unless your hair is absolutely filthy, there's no good reason to wash your hair twice, and it may

actually strip too many natural oils from your hair.

If it's a cloudy day at the beach, you don't need to wear sunscreen.

The sun's damaging UVA and UVB rays penetrate the clouds, and they can still damage your skin.

Sunscreen will protect my hair from sun damage.

The surface of your hair isn't flat, so it's almost impossible to get the coverage you'd need onto each and every hair. What you can do to keep hair soft and shiny after a day at the beach is to apply a leave-in conditioner, which helps prevent your hair from drying out and slows the sun from stripping color.

CHAPTER FIVE

Pregnancy and Postpartum

ES, A HEALTHY BABY IS THE MOST IMPORTANT thing, but what *you* look like along the way (and after you've given birth) is also a legitimate, healthy concern. After all, your hormones are over the moon, and the signs of turmoil will show up on your skin more than any other organ of the body.

Pregnancy can be a glorious time. Some women look (and feel) absolutely gorgeous (that rosy glow can be attributed to estrogen, which elevates your blood volume as much as 50 percent), while others can barely summon the energy to drag a comb through their ratty hair. For every woman who goes through pregnancy looking radiant, there's one who suffers from hyperpigmentation, dry skin, and acne. It's impossible to know whether your skin will glow and your hair will have incredible luster, or whether you'll break out like never before and lose small clumps of your crowning glory. Either way, rest assured, it will all revert back to normal.

Now is a great time to accentuate the positive. If you've suddenly got great cleavage, show off your décolleté with a pretty, plunging neckline. If your hair becomes luxurious and thick—most likely during your second trimester—splurge on a brand-new haircut or some stylish hair accessories. And if you're feeling large but your legs are lovely, flaunt them in a short skirt. Looking good and feeling sexy is important, not only during pregnancy, but also when you take on your new life-altering role as someone's mom. Here are some tips to ease your way through pregnancy and postpartum.

FACE

When your hormones are swinging, your face is the first place it shows. For some women, a glow comes naturally. Others may need to work at it. On the positive side, your blood volume rises and your skin may take on a healthy flush, your body retains water that plumps fine lines and wrinkles, and increased oil production may give you a nice, dewy look. But those hormones can also work in reverse and cause oiliness, puffiness, or dehydrated skin.

REGIME CHANGE

When you're pregnant, make these adjustments to your regime:

■ Wash your face with a gentle cleanser in the morning, at night, and after exercise (when you may be sweaty).

■ If you have breakouts, switch to a light oil-free moisturizer, which will hydrate your skin without clogging your pores.

■ Drink lots of water.

■ Change your pillowcase often to prevent breakouts.

BROKEN CAPILLARIES

Pregnancy—and the effort of childbirth—can burst small blood vessels and result in broken capillaries on the face. Massage a few drops of rose oil onto broken capillaries twice a day. Rose oil constricts small blood vessels and reduces redness. So does Visine.

PALE LIPS

Some pregnant women find that their natural lip color deepens; for others, it's a washout. If your lips pale and the idea—or smell—of lipstick sets your stomach churning, dip a wet Q-tip into cherry Jell-O powder and stroke it on your lips for a rosy stain.

WASHED OUT

Apply cream blush, bronzer, or powder with undertones of pink or gold.

PRODUCTS: Benefit Cosmetics Dandelion Powder ■ Lancôme Blush Papier Nacre ■ Agnes B. makeup.

SLEEPY TIME

You're tired, and it shows. The best way to get instant lift is to use an eyelash curler or curling mascara. Curly lashes draw attention upward.

SMUDGE-FREE FRINGE

Waterproof mascara can be hard to remove. To minimize that problem, first apply one coat of regular mascara, then top with a coat of waterproof mascara.

FAKE AWAKE

A dab of cheek gel on the apples of the cheeks is the best way to fake awake. Powder blush or foundation can make tired, dull skin look duller.

PRODUCTS: Bliss Ink Pink Blushing Balm ▪ Napoleon Barely Blushing Gel ▪ Clinique Gel Blush.

TIRED EYES

To look alert, stroke a light, neutral eye shadow over the top lid with a brush. Highlight your browbone with a pale shadow (or shimmer, for evening), which will also focus attention away from the droops.

EYE STRAIN

Keep the area underneath your eyes moist and supple with an eye cream.

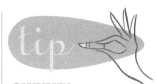

CHEEKY COLOR

Cheek gel often appears bright red in the tube, but it looks soft and rosy on your skin. Use just a dab and blend right away before it dries.

THE MASK OF PREGNANCY

Melasma, known as the mask of pregnancy, is most common in women of Asian and Hispanic descent, although it can affect anyone. Estrogen and progesterone stimulate melanin (pigment) in the skin, which causes dark blotches that look like a mask, mostly on the cheeks but sometimes on the chin, forehead, and lips. It fades after delivery, but in the meantime, avoid exposure to the sun. Use a sunscreen with SPF 15 and either titanium dioxide, zinc oxide, or avobenzene as an active ingredient.

Melasma is hard to treat during pregnancy, because some effective treatments such as hydrocortisone cream, Retin-A, skin bleaches, or lasers are not necessarily safe for pregnant women. Talk to your doctor, do your best to prevent it, and, if you get it, cover it up with concealer until after your baby is born and you're finished nursing.

BODY

It's hard to ignore your body right now, as it takes you through changes you could never have imagined. Weight gain, bloat, fatigue, itchy or scaly skin, and stretch marks are only a few. But some simple strategies can make you look—and feel—a whole lot better as you get ready to give birth, and beyond.

MOTHER'S MILK

It's important to drink a lot of water to keep you from dehydrating. Follow the example of my friend Peggy, who was most often found with baby Charlotte in one hand and a huge bottle of Evian in the other.

LIZARD SCALES

Moisturize, moisturize, moisturize. Apply moisturizer after you wash your face, after you shower, and whenever your skin feels tight or dry. Drink lots of water, and mist your face with water from a mini spray bottle. Avoid soap, and use a gentle cleanser instead.

SENSITIVE SKIN

Your skin will become more sensitive during pregnancy, and it may react negatively to certain products you've used, problem-free, for years. Switch to products that feature soothing, anti-inflammatory ingredients like chamomile and calendula.

PRODUCTS: Jurlique Calendula Cream ▪ California Baby Calendula Cream.

ITCHY SKIN

During the last trimester, some women suffer from pruritus gravidarum, an invisible itch throughout the body (most common on the abdomen). It's believed to be caused by a backup in the bile ducts. It will go away, but in the meantime, soak yourself in a cool colloidal bath (with oatmeal or Aveeno), and spritz or massage yourself with body oils, not creams or lotions.

PRODUCTS: Aveeno Anti-Itch Gel Spray ▪ Clarins Body Treatment Oil Tonic ▪ Soothing Care Itch Relief Spray.

HEY, SWEETIE

If your legs are dry and flaky—a common syndrome during pregnancy—take a handful of sugar, mix it with canola or sesame oil (sesame is one of the most absorbent oils), and massage into the skin before your bath or shower.

HOT AND SWEATY IN THE CITY

Keep a small spray bottle of water—or rose water—in your purse, and spritz as you go. Blot with a tissue, cotton bandanna, or handkerchief.

PRODUCTS: Eau Thermale Avène Thermal Water ▪ Shu Uemura Depsea Water.

TAG, YOU'RE IT!

In the second or third trimester, some women develop a tiny, raised growth of skin, especially in an area where friction is common, i.e., under the arm. It may go away after delivery. If not, a dermatologist can remove it easily. But to make sure that it's a skin tag and nothing that demands immediate attention, show it to your doctor.

FRECKLE NOT

Some women develop freckles when they're pregnant, especially if they spend time in the sun. Always use sunscreen with SPF 15. I think freckles look adorable, but if you don't:

▪ Massage freckles with fresh raw eggplant slices every day for a week, and see how they fade!

▪ Mix 2 teaspoons of fresh, grated horseradish with 2 tablespoons of buttermilk and refrigerate for a few hours. Strain out the horseradish, soak cotton pads in the liquid, and apply to freckled areas for five minutes. Then rinse well. Use twice a week for a few weeks.

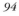

*What can I
do to avoid
stretch
marks?*

There is a way to
prevent stretch
marks, but it takes
diligence. Keep
your skin well
moisturized
when pregnant
(especially the
breasts, belly,
and hips)—by
slathering on an
absorbent oil
or rich cream
twice a day.

PRODUCTS: Kiehl's
Crème de Corps ▪
Clarins Body Treatment
Oil Tonic ▪ Jurlique
Calendula Cream ▪
Bliss Vanilla +
Bergamot Body Butter.

POLKA DOTS

Those mysterious red dots are called cherry hemangioma, caused by hormones and increased blood supply. They don't usually go away on their own, but you can have them lasered off after the pregnancy.

RED HANDED

Some women develop red, itchy palms, which return to normal after pregnancy. Meanwhile, apply a calendula cream (from the health-food store) to ease the condition. See "Sensitive Skin," page 234.

RASH ACTS

It's not uncommon to develop a red, bumpy, itchy rash on your stomach and thighs called PUPPP (pruritic urticarial papules and plaques of pregnancy). Consult your doctor for a topical cream to relieve itching.

DARK SPOTS

Some pregnant women find that their skin darkens (hyperpigmentation) in areas of the body that are darker already—the nipples, areola, genital area—and it happens in women of all races. It will go away when the baby is born, but if you find your skin continues to darken in more widespread areas, check with your doctor. It could indicate a hormonal problem that may need medical attention.

THIN BLACK LINE

The dark line that bisects the body in front, from the center of your abdomen to your pubic area, will go away when the baby is born. Sun exposure will make it worse. If it bothers you, apply concealer or cover it with body makeup.

PRODUCTS: M·A·C Face and Body Makeup ■ Dermablend Corrective Cosmetics Leg and Body Cover.

STRETCH MARKS

There's no way to completely eradicate stretch marks once you get them, but if you catch them in the early stages after delivery, when they're red or pink (in white women) or beige or tan (in darker-skinned women), a laser treatment at the dermatologist's office or Retin-A may be effective. Wait until you've

Pregnant Pause

VERY CLOSE VEINS

Even if you've never had varicose veins before, you may get them now. To minimize your chances:

■ Sleep on your left side if you can, because it will relieve pressure on the inferior vena cava, a vein on the right side of the body that circulates blood from the lower limbs to the heart. Elevate your feet slightly with a pillow.

■ Don't stand for too long without a rest.

■ Don't cross one leg over the other for extended periods of time.

■ Wear support hose.

■ Elevate your legs whenever you can.

■ Exercise every day to improve your circulation—even a short walk will help.

STYLISH SHORTCUT

If your maternity wardrobe is limited, and you've hand-washed a special shirt or pair of jeans that's not quite dry, give it a few blasts with your blow-dryer, and it will be good to go in no time.

stopped breast-feeding. Or, massage a rich cream or gel into new stretchmarks twice a day for a month.

PRODUCTS: StriVectin SD ■ Sothys Freshening Gel.

SECOND TRIMESTER BLOAT

It's not unusual to feel bloated around your second or third trimester. Your entire face—or the area under your eyes—may puff up like a blowfish! Keep a bottle of alcohol-free toner in the refrigerator. Apply it to two cotton pads, tilt your head back, close your eyes, and place the cotton pads on your eyes. Relax for ten minutes, and when you arise, you'll be a lot less bloated.

DOWN DOGS

Put a removable gel insert in the sole of your sandals to cushion the blow and put the spring back in your step. Also, soak or scrub your feet with a mint product. Mint refreshes, invigorates, and tingles the tootsies!

PRODUCTS: Airplus for Her Invisigel ■ Bliss Super Minty Soap 'n Scrub ■ Essencia Rosemary Mint Body Polish.

WEIGHT-BEARING LOAD

Just because you can't see your legs doesn't mean you don't want to feel them. Legs that support pregnancy's heavy load can become overheated and almost numb with exhaustion. Try one of these.

PRODUCTS: Kneipp Arnica Active Spray ■ Clarins Energizing Emulsion.

SORE NIPPLES

It's normal to feel nipple soreness when you first start to nurse, but it shouldn't last more than a few days. Alternate the baby's position when you nurse. When you're done, break the suction first by gently removing the baby's mouth from your nipple with your finger before you pull the baby from your breast.

To relieve pain, massage some of your breast milk onto your nipples every time you nurse; it soothes them and helps them to heal. Or, apply Lansinoh or PureLan to your nipples—these lanolin creams are considered safe for babies. Beware of over-the-counter products that contain antibiotics, steroids, anesthetics, fragrances, or colorants, which are not safe for your baby. Wear nipple pads—available at the drugstore—to lessen the friction against your bra, and wear a cotton bra. If your nipples remain cracked for more than a few days, check with your doctor. You may be at risk for an infection.

CHIPPY NAILS

Your nails will probably grow faster—especially around the fourth month—but they can also become soft or brittle. To prevent chipping, apply a stroke of clear hardener under your nails when you polish, and sweep the applicator brush against the absolute edge of the nail.

WEAK NAILS

Strengthen nails by soaking them in warm olive oil for ten minutes every other day. Give your nails a beveled edge by buffing them up and down with a nail buffer.

DULL NAILS

Apply cuticle oil to nails (and cuticles) and buff with a chamois cloth.

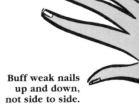

Buff weak nails up and down, not side to side.

prenatal yoga

If you practice yoga, even on an occasional basis, you'll have a more comfortable pregnancy. Look for classes taught by instructors trained in prenatal yoga. If they're not available in your area, make sure that your instructor is experienced with pregnant women, and make sure to tell him or her that you are pregnant.

Yoga strengthens the abdominal muscles, which can relieve back pain; alleviates sciatica and leg cramps through stretching; stimulates circulation, which can increase your energy; and stretches the pelvic area to help prepare for childbirth. Plus, it's great for your posture. Your breasts get heavy during pregnancy, and the normal tendency is to slump. Yoga opens up the chest and elongates the spine.

Stretching increases flexibility, which comes in really handy as the pregnancy progresses. When you're flexible, you get around more easily and don't feel as tired as you would if your muscles were tight. It's important to take precautions with any exercise program, especially when you are pregnant. Here are a few important guidelines:

Yoga invigorates the body and soothes the mind.

■ **Avoid deep twists and back-bends**, which can strain and possibly tear the abdominal muscles and create more pressure on the lower back.

■ **Avoid positions that require you to lie on your back** after the first trimester, unless you're supported by bolsters or blankets at a 45-degree angle or higher. Holding a supine position may put too much pressure on your inferior vena cava, cutting off the blood supply from the legs to the heart and causing dizziness.

■ **Lying on your belly is not a good idea**, especially in the third trimester, for obvious reasons.

■ Unless you're experienced in yoga, **avoid the plank pose**, which can create too much sway in your back.

■ If you're not an advanced yogi, it's important to **stay away from inverted poses** like headstands and shoulder stands. The extra weight of your pregnancy puts too much pressure on your neck and can put you at greater risk of injury.

■ **Avoid poses that require balancing on your arms** (like the crow pose). Pregnant women are more prone to carpal tunnel syndrome, and arm balances will make that worse.

■ **Don't hold poses for too long**, especially in the second trimester, when your joints are loosening.

■ **Move into poses slowly** to avoid injury.

FAKE FRENCH MANICURE

If you'd rather not breathe in noxious fumes from nail polish, fake it: Massage cuticle oil onto nails, then stroke a white nail pencil (or eye pencil) under each nail tip.

HAIR TODAY, GONE TOMORROW

A surge in androgens—sex hormones— may cause the growth of new hair on your upper lip, chin, breasts, belly, or maybe even cheeks and back, especially during your first trimester. It will go away within three to six months after the birth of your baby, but if you want to get rid of it before then, wax.

SCALY SPOTS

Use an old toothbrush to exfoliate dry, flaky knees and elbows. Apply moisturizer first, and gently massage it in with the toothbrush.

A well-manicured look without the potential health risks.

HAIR

Your hair may act as schizophrenic as you feel: formerly sleek, shiny straight hair seems to transform itself virtually overnight into a cloud of frizz. Thick, voluminous curls suddenly go limp and lose their body. It will all eventually return to normal, but in the meantime, follow good hair care techniques and choose good products. Treat your hair gently, minimize heat styling, and avoid coloring or perming your hair during this time.

SCARE HAIR

Static can be a sign of dry hair. Dab a tiny, tiny bit of sweet almond oil on your palm, pat palms together, and pat through your hair.

POSTPARTUM FUZZY-WUZZY

Even women with straight, sleek hair sometimes find their hair reinvents itself as soon as they stop nursing. It can turn into a dry, frizzy mess. Until it gets back to normal, use a moisturizing shampoo and conditioner along with a good haircut.

PRODUCTS: L'Oreal Nature's Therapy Unfrizz Treatment ■ Kerastase Lait Vital Protein Conditioner ■ Infusium 23 Power Pac Revitalizing Conditioner.

STYLE-RESISTANT FRIZZ

If your hair frizzes when you try to style it, use a good defrizzing styling aid.

PRODUCTS: Kerastase Oleo Relax ■ KMS Back to Lift Hair Cream.

MAKING WAVES

Make chunky braids around your head before bed. Unbraid and scrunch mousse through in the a.m.

HAIR COLOR

Most doctors now consider hair-coloring safe after the first trimester. But if you're concerned, stick with henna or high-lights. (In highlighting, the foil reduces contact of your scalp with chemicals.)

Now that I've given birth, I seem to be losing my hair. Is that normal?

We all lose around 70 hairs every day, but hormones keep most pregnant women from losing that hair. It's got to go eventually, and, most often, hair loss occurs within three to six months after you've had your baby or after you stop breast-feeding. Take a multiple vitamin supplement. Don't worry. It will all grow back.

is it safe?

No matter how much you love to try new skincare products, it's not the time when you're pregnant or nursing your baby. The skin is extremely absorbent, and you'll want to make sure that whatever you put on your hair, skin, and nails is not going to put you or your baby at risk. It's always smart to check with your ob/gyn before signing on for a salon or spa treatment, and ask about the safety of your beauty products as well. Also, check with your dermatologist or ob/gyn if your skin or hair condition radically changes during pregnancy. Here's a guide to some red flags.

Acne medication

Avoid prescription acne medications like Accutane (extremely dangerous to the developing fetus), Retin-A, Differin, and Tazorac, which can pose a high risk of birth defects.

Antiaging treatments

Avoid. If you're an older mom, now's the time to take a break from Botox, Retin-A, and other topical vitamin A treatments.

Aromatherapy spa treatments

Some essential oils may be harmful during pregnancy, so be cautious before signing on for an aromatherapy spa treatment. Avoid the following oils, which may stimulate contractions of the uterus: rosemary, sage, thyme, clary sage, marjoram, myrrh, basil, fennel, cedarwood, and juniper.

Depilatories

Avoid—they can be absorbed into the skin, and it's not known how they affect the developing baby.

Glycolics

Avoid glycolic acids, salicylic acids, and alpha and beta hydroxy acids, which can irritate sensitive skin and may trigger hyperpigmentation during pregnancy—or make it worse.

Reflexology treatments

Avoid, unless your reflexologist is extremely skilled and experienced in working with pregnant women. Reflexology is a treatment where pressure is applied to certain points on the feet (and ears and hands), intended to stimulate energy flow throughout the body. But pressure on the wrong points can stimulate contractions.

Soy-based moisturizers that reduce hair growth

Avoid—they may contain plant hormones.

Hot baths

Take warm—not hot—baths or showers. Excessively hot water can dry the skin and may raise your body temperature, making it unhealthy for the baby.

Hot tubs

Avoid. Soaking in water that significantly increases the body temperature for more than ten minutes is not a good idea in the first few months of pregnancy because it can put the baby at risk for neural tube defects. Don't worry if you've already had a soak, but exercise caution before you do it again.

Mud baths and body wraps

Not a good idea, because your body temperature rises significantly.

Self-tanner

Probably okay, since the chemicals that trigger the tan are restricted to the top layers of the skin, but there's no hard evidence either way.

Nail polish

Go ahead, but make sure that your manicure and pedicure is done in a well-ventilated space so that you breathe in as few strong chemicals as possible.

Perms

Avoid, because your hair responds unpredictably when you're pregnant. Your perm may turn into frizz, or it may not take at all. And, the perm chemicals can be absorbed into the bloodstream. Though no conclusive link has been found between perms and birth defects, it's best to err on the side of caution.

Hair relaxing

The jury is out. There's no evidence that hair relaxing is dangerous, and no proof that it's safe. And, as with perms, there's no guarantee that your hair will take to the process, anyway.

Tattooing

Avoid. This is not the time—the risk of infection through unsterilized needles is just not worth it.

Massage

Go for it—but preferably not during your first trimester, when you may get dizzy and make your morning sickness worse. Check that the massage therapist is fully licensed and experienced with pregnancy massage. Do not massage the feet, ankles, or tissue between the thumb and index finger—certain points in those spots can trigger contractions.

CHAPTER SIX

Menopause
and Aging

MENOPAUSE CAN LEAD TO ALL KINDS OF MOOD swings on the inside and beauty meltdowns on the outside. Between the ages of 45 to 55, most women secrete less estrogen, release fewer eggs, and begin to have irregular periods—a stage known as perimenopause. When you haven't had your period for a year, you've officially entered menopause (the average age for American women is 51).

Lowered estrogen levels slow the skin's normal functions. Hot flashes can cause sudden sweats and make it hard to sleep through the night, resulting in dark circles below the eyes. Your skin becomes dry and flaky; the face can look drawn and sag. In some women, facial hair—especially around the lip and chin—can sprout out of nowhere due to the increase in male hormones. You're hot and bothered, cold and clammy, moody and irritable, and not exactly feeling gorgeous, either!

Who has time for this? You do, because in spite of all these challenges, the middle years and beyond can be the most beautiful of your life. What you may have lost in estrogen, you've gained in wisdom and self-knowledge, and that's reflected in your face. The beauty industry may still focus its efforts on youth—though that is changing—but you are becoming a stronger, even more beautiful version of who you truly are. However, it still helps to know how to deal with the more common signs of aging (and the fallout from some antiaging procedures, if you so choose to go that route).

FACE

Since older skin doesn't shed cells as quickly, and new ones don't grow as fast, the skin can start to look dull as we age. Collagen and elastin lose their snap, the fat layer thins and the skin can lose some of its firmness. But making a few tweaks to your skincare regimen—and some simple quick fixes—can make a big difference.

GOOD STUFF

When Lauren Hutton launched her makeup line for midlife women, called Good Stuff, she was asked, "What's bad about aging?" and she replied, "You have less energy and strength." When asked, "What's good?" she said, "You learn how to spend your strength where it counts!"

Better As You Get Older

After 50, your skin isn't able to retain moisture as well, it produces less oil, and it becomes dryer, flakier, and ashier. Switch to a creamy cleanser and a richer moisturizer, exfoliate your skin more frequently, use a moisturizing mask once a week, and tweak your makeup. See if any of these small changes make a big difference for you.

Yes	No
Lighter, sheerer shades	Dark lipstick
Charcoal, brown, or navy	Black eyeliner
Mascara on top lashes only	Mascara on lower lashes
Lip crayon (moisturizing)	Lip pencil
Lipstick or gloss applied like a stain	Lip liner
Sunscreen	Suntan
Pale pink, neutral, or color nail polish	Brown, taupe, frosty nail polish
Soft, swingy styles	helmet hair
Cream or gel blush	Powder blush

FAST FREEZE

To put a temporary freeze on lines under the eyes, try an eye cream with peptides, which smooth lines for a few hours.

PRODUCTS: L'Oréal Eye Wrinkle Decrease ■ Freeze 24/7 Ice Cream.

LINE PLUMPER

To soften the little lines on your face, put a bit of moisturizer—Lubriderm lotion works especially well—on your fingers to warm it up and, after you apply foundation, pat it between the nose and chin, under eyes, or anywhere you have lines and want to soften them.

ROAD BURN

Avoid powder formulations that are apt to streak on dry skin. Instead, look for creamy foundation, eye shadow, and lipstick. Apply moisturizer before you apply foundation, and give it a minute to sink in. Or, mix moisturizer with foundation in your palm, then apply to your face.

THIN LIPS

To make thin lips fuller, draw a thick line on your lips with lip crayon, and blend it in toward the center of the mouth with your fingers. Apply gloss in the center of the top and bottom lips, and extend it out toward the edges with your fingers. Make sure to keep the color even, which adds fullness to the lips.

I'm noticing frown lines on my brows, but I'm not up for Botox. What can I do?

To ease wrinkles in a less invasive way, try one of the topical creams known as "Botox in a bottle." The active ingredients —peptides— are high-tech amino acids said to soften lines caused by repeated facial movements. They will make you look better—for a few hours.

PRODUCTS: Therapy Systems Line Tox ■ Dr. Brandt Crease Release ■ DDF Wrinkle Relax ■ Olay Regenerist Daily Regenerating Serum ■ StriVectin SD.

CHEEK LIFT

When you apply blush, don't get too close to the lines that run from the bottom of your nose to the corners of your lips. It will emphasize the lines. Keep your blush high, around the apples of your cheeks, to create a look of "lift" in your face.

SMILE LINES

If it's been a long day, and your lines loom large, plump them up: dip a makeup sponge into moisturizing lotion, and dab it over the area, smoothing it out on top of your makeup.

PASSING POUT

To plump your lips, try lip plumpers with niacin, a form of vitamin B that pumps up the circulation, which plumps up the lips.

PRODUCTS: Alex and Ani Serious Lip Plump ▪ Freeze 24/7 Plump Lips ▪ Joey New York Super Duper Lips ▪ L'Oréal Two-Sided Volume Perfect Lipcolour.

LIP BLEED

It gets harder to keep lipstick where it belongs, especially if you wear deep pigments like burgundy or red. To keep your lipstick in line, take a pointed lip brush and stroke a small amount of translucent powder just outside the edges of your lips before you apply lipstick.

LIP LINES

To touch up and cover lines above the lips, use a concealer pencil around your lips. (You can also try your regular concealer, but if it mixes with your lipstick, it can change the color.)

PRODUCTS: Agnes B. Crayon Anti-Cernes ▪ Sephora Cooling Cover Stick ▪ Darphin Concealer Pencil ▪ Estée Lauder Perfectionist Correcting Concentrate for Lip Lines.

LESS LIP

Sometimes it seems our lips are the only things that do get thinner. To create the look of more lip, try a lighter, neutral lip shade in a cream formulation with a hint of shimmer.

CRINKLY LIPS

Avoid matte lipstick. Apply creamy color in the form of a lip crayon. For just a hint of color with shine, mix lip balm in your palm with a few strokes from the crayon, and press it into your lips with fingers.

THE SKIN YOU'RE IN

For aging skin that's acting out, look for these ingredients to rein it in.

PROBLEM	INGREDIENTS TO LOOK FOR
Dullness	Seaweed and algae, papaya enzymes, kinetin, soy, alpha or beta hydroxy acid, lactic or glycolic acid, copper peptide, retinoids, L-ascorbic acid (vitamin C).
Dark spots	Kojic acid, licorice extract (a.k.a. glycyrrhizinate).
Sagging skin	Hyaluronic acid, soy, copper peptide, L-ascorbic acid.
Lines and wrinkles	Plant oils, peptides, green tea, kinetin, retinols (vitamin A derivatives), L-ascorbic acid, DMAE, seaweed and algae, hyaluronic acid.
Breakouts (adult acne)	Tea tree oil, parsley, lycopene (from tomatoes), citrus, mint, rosemary, retinols, salicylic acid, sulfur, resorcinol, glycolic acid, which works to fight acne as well as aging.
Blotchiness, redness, irritation	Cucumber, aloe, chamomile, green tea, licorice extract (a.k.a. glycyrrhizinate).

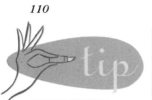

SENSITIVE EYES

If your eyes have gotten too sensitive for eye makeup, try mineral makeup. It has no irritating additives, which is why cosmetic surgeons recommend it post-surgery.

PRODUCTS: Bare Escentuals ■ Jane Ireland Mineral Make-up ■ Pur Minerals ■ Colorscience ■ Glo Minerals.

SMUDGES

If you've been thinking about eyelash tinting because your mascara smudges and you can't stand it anymore—especially with hot flashes—switch your mascara first. Try Kiss Me Mascara by Blinc, formulated to coat each lash individually and stay there. When you wash it off, press your lashes gently, and the casings release into the sink.

LOSING LASHES

If you start to lose lashes, try this French import: Talika Lipocils lash conditioner. Sounds impossible, but they actually grow back—soft and lush as ever. And remember: No matter how tired you are, never go to bed with your eye makeup on.

HOT SPOTS

To cover red spots or spotty discoloration—not uncommon as we get older—apply cream foundation or stick concealer to those areas with a medium-size brush, and blend the color into your skin really well. Use gentle strokes, so as not to pull dry skin.

FLASH POINTS

To calm a hot-flash-related splotch or red flush on your face, neck or chest, try one of these anti-inflammatory creams.

PRODUCTS: Clinique CX Redness Relief Cream ■ Eucerin Redness Relief Daily Perfecting Lotion ■ Therapy Systems Emergency Treatment Cream ■ Origins Constant Comfort.

RUDDY PATINA

Apply translucent powder in a banana shade over your foundation to tone down the red. For an even dusting, apply powder to a drugstore powder puff, then press it onto your face.

PRODUCTS: T. LeClerc Pressed Powder Banane ■ Bobbi Brown Pressed Powder (pale yellow).

DISAPPEARING EYES

Dab a bit of pale, buttery eye shadow under the arches of the brows to make the eyes pop.

SALLOW SKIN

A bit of cheek gel or cream blush gives a healthy, natural flush to the skin, and if you put a tiny bit on the browbone, it will warm the entire face.

MAKEUP LOOKS SPACKLED

Apply and blend foundation with a *dry* makeup sponge for a natural look. If you want a thinner application, dampen the sponge.

WARM UP

To make your eyes stand out, and to warm up dull skin, ask your colorist about balliage—painting strands of hair around the face in a lighter shade to complement your hair color, without the use of foils. It adds dimension to the hair and helps frame and warm the face.

BARGAIN BINS

The beauty department of a super-size drugstore can be dizzying, which is why you may miss some great bargain skincare brands. More European skincare companies are entering the mass marketplace in the U.S., which is a good thing for consumers. Look for French imports RoC, Yves Rocher, and Eau Thermale Avene, along with Scandinavian stand-out Lumene.

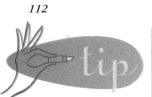

MAKEUP ARTISTS' TRICK

To deflect the light away from dark circles, try a dab of Chanel Blanc Universel de Chanel Sheer Illuminator or Laura Mercier Secret Brightener on top of your concealer. These stark white products may look scary in the package, but they look soft and subtle on the face.

SLIPPERY CONCEALER

When you're having hot flashes, your concealer can slip into the lines under your eyes. To avoid, try a brush-on concealer (from a pen applicator), a lightweight product with heavy-duty coverage that won't slip.

PRODUCTS: Clinique Airbrush Concealer ■ Laura Mercier Secret Brightener ■ Yves Saint Laurent Touche Eclat ■ Neutrogena SkinClearing Oil Free Concealer.

FADE OUT

To emphasize your disappearing eyes, take a brown—not black—eye pencil, and press the color as close to the lash line as possible for a strong but natural look. (Black may look too severe as you get older.)

WAXING WOES

Glycolic acids and chemical peels can make the face extra sensitive to waxing. If you use them regularly on your face, tweeze your brows instead of waxing.

PEELED LIKE A GRAPE

To calm your skin down after a chemical peel or laser treatment, try these.

PRODUCTS: Clinique CX Rapid Recovery Cream ■ Aquaphor Healing Ointment ■ Eau Thermale Avène Soothing Serum.

BOTOX BRUISES

A side effect of Botox and other injections may be bruising, caused by broken blood vessels from the needle puncture. To correct, apply cold compresses to constrict blood vessels, and a topical vitamin K cream (a.k.a. phytonadione).

PRODUCTS: St. Ives Vitamin K Dark Circle Diminisher ▪ Reviva Labs Vitamin K Cream ▪ Jason Naturals Vitamin K Creme Plus.

DULL NIGHT

For an evening warm-up, dab a shimmer blush or highlighter on your cheekbones and browbones. It will make you look well lit from within—even when you don't feel that way.

PRODUCTS: Nars Gold Member Cream Blush ▪ Delux Beauty Glistener Highlighter.

DULL GIRL

Sweep out the dead-skin buildup and debris with a super-exfoliating treatment, which will perk up your dull, aging skin.

PRODUCTS: Estée Lauder Idealist Micro-D ▪ Prescriptives Dermapolish Treatment Cream ▪ Bliss Steep Clean ▪ Good Skin All Bright Step Facial Peel Pads.

CLEANUP CREW

When the skin around your eyes is dry, it can be harder to remove your eye makeup without tugging, which you *don't* want to do. Try these gentle but muscular eye-makeup removers.

PRODUCTS: Talika Oil-Free Lash Conditioning Cleanser ▪ Clinique Rinse-Off Eye Makeup Solvent ▪ Clarins Gentle Eye Make-Up Remover Lotion.

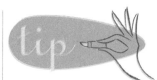

FLASHING

Keep a cup of mint tea chilled in the fridge to take down the heat. Moisten a washcloth in the tea, squeeze, and press around your face for a couple of minutes. Pour the excess in a mini spray bottle. Carry it in your purse, and spray your face (blotting with a tissue) throughout the day.

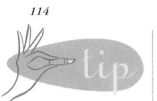

LASTING VALUE

Firming creams can be pricey. To make yours last longer, mix a little bit in with your regular moisturizer.

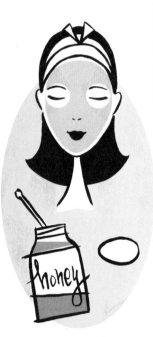

SAGGING SKIN

Try a firming cream. The results, though fleeting, can tighten up the look of your skin. An ingredient to look for is hyaluronic acid, which binds moisture into the skin, or soy proteins or soy isoflavones.

PRODUCTS: RoC Protein Lift Daily Firming Moisturizer ■ Kerstin Florian Caviar Firming Complex ■ Lancome Renergie Microlift ■ Kinerase Cream.

EYE PROTECTION

When you wear eye makeup after cosmetic surgery, only use brand-new makeup and fresh applicators to avoid infection. During the first few months, you may want to try mineral makeup, which has no potentially irritating chemicals or additives.

LOSING YOUR SNAP

For temporary tightening of the face when you want to play Cinderella for a night, try one of these:

■ Apply tomato juice, preferably squeezed from a fresh tomato, to clean skin for ten minutes. Rinse with cool water.

■ Mix one egg white with 2 tablespoons honey. Apply to the face and leave on for ten minutes. Rinse with warm, then cool water.

PRODUCTS: Clinique Anti-Gravity Firming Lift Mask ■ Dior Capture R Flash Instant Ultra Smoothing Fluid ■ Chantecaille Biodynamic Lifting Cream.

OLD YELLAH

Bleaching is probably your best option for whitening teeth. It takes an hour or two with a "super" bleach or "power" bleach at your dentist's. Your dentist can also fit you for a custom "take home" bleaching system, which takes anywhere from two to four weeks. Or, try an at-home whitening system yourself.

PRODUCT: Go Smile Advanced Bl (seven days).

SAGGING SMILE

As we age, our teeth change. They discolor, the gums thin (which can make your teeth look less even), and your teeth can shift, which may alter the shape of your face and make you look older. If you notice a change, consult your dentist. In many cases, cosmetic dentistry—from tooth whitening to tooth shaping to realignment—is a lot less invasive than cosmetic surgery.

COLOR CARE

Brighter shades of lipstick emphasize lines and wrinkles, especially around the eyes; soft, neutral shades downplay them.

MAKEUP SLIDE

In the heat of a hot flash, your makeup can slide off your face. Look for creamy products with extra staying power.

PRODUCTS: Clinique Workout All-Day Wear Makeup ■ L'Oréal Cashmere Perfect ■ Chantecaille Real Skin.

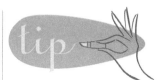

CREASY EYE SHADOW

If oily eye shadow collects in the creases of your lids, brush a bit of powder over the lids after you apply cream shadow. Or, try these eye shadows, which won't smudge.

PRODUCTS: Sue Devitt Starlights Clear Water Eye Shadow ■ Laura Mercier Cream Eye Color.

the eyes have it

Dark shadows Insomnia may not take all the blame for your creature-of-the-night gaze. If you spend too many of your waking hours surfing eBay or staring at the television, or if you are genetically predisposed to undereye circles, here's what to do:

To get rid of them:

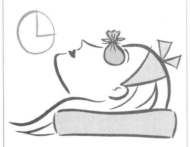

■ Wrap a bit of grated raw potato in cheesecloth or slice a kiwi. Lie down, and apply to eye area for 15 minutes. Pat dry.

■ Look for eye creams with vitamin K (phytonadione), used by cosmetic surgeons because it prevents bruising, peptides, or kinetin.

PRODUCTS: St. Ives Vitamin K Dark Circle Diminisher ■ K-Derm gel ■ Kinerase Intensive Eye Cream ■ Hylexin ■ Clarins Bright Plus Target Zone Corrector.

To conceal them:

■ Avoid plum, purple, and red shades of eye shadow. You'll look like you've got two black eyes.

■ Try a concealer with a pink, peachy, or yellow undertone to neutralize the blue and green in the circles under your eyes.

■ Look for light-reflecting concealers that downplay dark circles.

PRODUCTS: Prescriptives Vibrant Instant Eye Brightener ■ L'Oréal Visible Lift Eye Line Minimizing Concealer ■ Bourjois Light Reflective Liquid Concealer ■ Laura Mercier Undercover.

TIP: *When the circles are really dark, take a tiny bit of creamy white eye shadow and dab it in the corners of the eyelids, top and bottom. (If you're dark-skinned, use a light brown shade.) Blend well, then apply concealer on top and around the eyes.*

PUFFY EYES Don't *look* tired—even if you feel it.

The night before:

■ Cut back on salt and drink a glass of water before bed. Use an extra pillow to keep your head elevated when you sleep.

■ Pat a chilled eye gel on the area.

■ Use products with anti-inflammatory ingredients like chamomile, green tea, or antioxidants. Drink Gatorade, or sports drinks with electrolytes, which help deflate puffs.

PRODUCTS: Origins No Puffery Gel ■ Chanel Precision Age Delay Eye ■ Jurlique Eye Gel ■ Kimberly Sayer of London Cellular Extract Eye Lift Gel.

The morning after:

■ Keep two spoons in the freezer. Lie down with the bowl of a spoon over each eye for five minutes.

■ Lie down with a small flaxseed-, buckwheat- or lavender-filled pillow over the eyes. Or, place some rice in a zippered plastic bag, refrigerate until chilled, lie down, and hold over the eyes.

■ Dip a washcloth in a bowl of cool, caffeinated coffee. Apply to the area, and leave on for ten minutes. Caffeine is a diuretic, which means that it draws water away.

■ Sit down, lean forward, and hold your face in your hands for a couple of minutes; the pressure will help you depuff.

■ Try a portable depuffing eye mask. Pop one in the hotel minibar to help chill out from jet lag, or keep it in the fridge at home when you need to soothe tired eyes. These also take down surgery-related swelling.

■ Try a stick-on undereye patch infused with gels and plant extracts like chamomile, cucumber, mint, and aloe. Chill in the fridge overnight, and apply for ten minutes in the morning.

PRODUCTS: Talika Eye Therapy Patch ■ Chanel Precision Eye Patch Total ■ Earth Therapeutics Hydrogel Under-Eye Recovery Patch ■ Pearl Ice Cooling Mask by Inka.

TIP: *Eyeliner and a too-light concealer can draw attention to puffs; draw the focus away from the eye area with blush and lipstick.*

HAIR

It's not unusual for your hair to thin, change texture, and get drier as you grow older, especially if you've spent years processing your hair, and your hormones are acting out. If the situation continues to worsen, consult a cosmetic dermatologist. Otherwise, look for moisturizing shampoos, conditioners, hair masks, and salon treatments that will put the silky softness back into your hair.

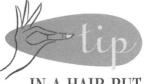

IN A HAIR RUT

Changing your hairstyle can provide a nice boost. But why does your hair always look ten times better when you leave the salon than when you do it yourself? Next time, put the magazine down and watch your stylist. Ask her to show you exactly how to style it yourself.

BROKEN HAIR

If your hair is broken off around your face, comb a bit of gel through your hair with your fingers, which will distribute the product lightly and evenly, and slick down those messy pieces.

STRAY GRAYS

When you start to see a few stragglers—or more than a few—highlighting is an attractive, low-maintenance way to go. Even when the gray grows back, it won't attract as much attention as it would with a single-process color. At-home highlighting kits are an inexpensive option, but don't try them unless you're really competent or have a friend over who is (think about what the back will look like!).

YOUR ROOTS ARE SHOWING

Touch up gray roots with black or brown mascara, and brush through with an eyelash brush or old toothbrush. If you're blond, dip a clean mascara wand or spoolie into your foundation, and brush it on your roots. Or, wet an eye shadow brush and brush on a complementary shade of eye shadow.

PRODUCT: Clairol Nice 'n Easy Root Touch-Up.

PERM CONTROL

If your hair is damaged by perms, don't go back for more. Consider a great haircut. You'll be surprised at how easy it is to build in a more textured, swingy look by cutting a few layers into your hair and gradating the length.

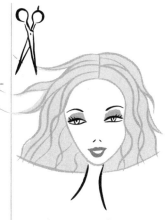

Make sure your layers are blended, not choppy.

THINNING HAIR

One in four women suffer from thinning hair after the age of 50—that's about 35 million women. No matter what the cause—chemical abuse, aggressive manual styling, poor diet, unhealthy habits, genetics, or hormonal changes—thinning hair inevitably leads to anxiety, feelings of insecurity, even depression. Besides bringing out the heavy artillery—prescription medication or Rogaine, which often yield good results—here's what you can do to prevent breakage and help hold on to what's left.

▓ Gently massage the scalp while you hold your head upside down, once or twice a day to increase blood flow to the roots.

▓ Avoid heavy styling products and shampoos that weigh the hair down.

▓ Don't condition your scalp, which can clog pores and inhibit hair growth.

▓ Try volumizing shampoos that make the most of the hair that you have and help each strand look thicker.

▓ Be sure to take multivitamins in case it's a nutritional deficiency.

▓ Avoid styles that pull the hair too tightly.

PRODUCTS: Pantene Full and Thick Shampoo ▓ Nioxin.

OVER-DRIED AND REFRIED

Slick a deep, moisturizing conditioner through dry hair. Leave on for about ten to 15 minutes, and it will absorb into your hair. Shampoo, condition, rinse, and style. This "hair mask" will help to soften and moisturize the hair in the same way that a face mask gives extra oomph to your face.

TAKE A SHINE TO IT

Put a dab of body oil in your palms, pat hands together, and pat on dry hair.

STRAY GRAY BROWS

Do not pluck, pull, or otherwise mutilate your poor gray stragglers. It will leave your brows looking spotty. Try a tinted brow gel until you're ready to go gray or color your brows along with your hair.

Body oil conditions, softens, and adds shine to hair.

PRODUCTS: Benefit Cosmetics Speed Brow ■ CG Smoothers Cover Girl Natural Lash and Brow Mascara ■ Paula Dorf Brow Tint Eyebrow Gel.

WHITER WHITES

If you want to get the yellow out and brighten the white, try laundry bluing— seriously! Dilute 1 teaspoon in a half-quart of warm water. Use as a final rinse after you shampoo.

PRODUCTS: Aveda Blue Malva Color Conditioner ■ Phyto Phytargent Whitening Shampoo.

BODY

Though you may not look as good as Teri Hatcher or Jane Fonda (who does?), if you exercise regularly (even a daily walk helps!) and eat a healthy diet rich in fruits, vegetables, and protein, your body should still look good as you get older. Here's how to fix the little things that come up along the way.

SPIDER VEINS

To camouflage spider veins, mix a heavy cream foundation with a tiny dab of body lotion, and pat gently back and forth over the veins.

PRODUCTS: M·A·C Face and Body Foundation ■ Dermablend Coverage Cosmetics Cover Creme.

BAGGY KNEES

The skin around the knees—frequently exposed on the tennis or golf course—is especially vulnerable to sagging. Strengthen the quadricep muscles above the knees to make the skin look more taut. Knee bends, squats, or the table position in yoga, two or three times a week, will help tighten up and tone your knees. Then don't forget the sunscreen!

DARK SPOTS

Skin-lightening products with soy proteins, vitamin A, kojic acid, or licorice extracts (glycyrrhizinates) will fade spots, but it takes at least three or four weeks. (If extensive, consult a dermatologist, who may

FLEX THOSE MUSCLES!

By your mid-40s, you're likely to lose a quarter pound of muscle each year and gain that much in body fat. That's one reason why it's so important to keep up some form of weight-bearing exercise—and walking counts. Aerobic and strengthening exercises can completely reverse the fat gain/muscle loss equation—and strengthen bone mass, which one out of two women begin to lose after the age of 50.

*Is there
anything
to do for
cellulite?*

There's no magic
pill for cellulite,
but determina-
tion and a good
massage brush
may slowly break
it down. Apply a
body moisturizer
to the hip and
thigh area, then
brush vigorously
for five minutes
every day. It's the
massage action,
not the product,
that helps. Or,
roll a rolling pin
over your hips
and thighs for
about five min-
utes each day.

recommend laser treatments, dermabrasion, or prescription topical treatments.)

PRODUCTS: MD Formulations Vit-a-Plus Illuminating Serum ■ Dr. Brandt Lightening Gel ■ Shiseido Whiteness Intensive Skin Brightener ■ RoC Age Diminishing Daily Moisturizer.

SCALY SKIN

Mix equal parts honey and sugar, and gently scrub on arms, legs, and torso. Or use an exfoliating body scrub in the shower. Rinse with warm water.

ROUGH ELBOWS AND KNEES

Extra-tough spots like elbows, knees, and heels may need extra-strength exfolia-tion. Apply a glycolic acid body lotion before bed, and wake up with slinkier skin.

PRODUCTS: Therapy Systems Glycolic Body Treatment ■ MD Formulations Glycare Lotion.

LACKLUSTER SKIN

For dull-looking skin, get instant results with an exfoliating mask.

PRODUCTS: Naturopathica Environmental Defense Mask ■ Astara Activated Sea Mineral Mask.

CREPEY CHEST

The chest has very thin skin, and it needs extra moisture—especially during and after menopause. For an intensive moisturiz-ing treatment, apply body oil to the chest and neck first, then seal it with a rich, unscented lotion or cream. Buyer Beware: Products that are labeled "fragrance free" sometimes contain scent.

PRODUCT: Osea Ocean Lotion (unscented).

STICK YOUR NECK OUT

No, you don't have to wear turtlenecks! Make sure to apply sun protection to your neck (and hands) in addition to your face, and moisturize. Try a moisturizer with kinetin—a gentle, plant-based exfoliating agent—or soy for aging skin on face and neck.

PRODUCTS: Almay Kinetin Age Decelerating Daily Cream ■ Osmotics Kinetin Cellular Renewal Serum ■ Kinerase ■ Lancôme Absolue.

HANDS DOWN

Why do we carefully coat our faces with SPF, but forget about our hands? Hands that come into contact with the sun's UV rays are usually the first to reveal age. Look for a hand cream with SPF 15—and use it. Or, when you're applying sunscreen to your face, wipe the excess from your palms onto the backs of your hands.

PRODUCT: Boscia Daily Hand Revival Therapy SPF 15.

MOODY BLUES

When your moods are really swinging, sit yourself down and get a grip. Mix a few drops of essential oil (lavender is calming, mint is a pick-me-up) with an inexpensive body lotion like Nivea or Lubiderm in

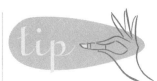

TIME OUT

When you need to take a pause from your busy, stressful, overcommitted life, light an aromatherapy candle. (The soy versions burn longer and are cleaner than most.)

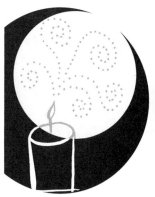

your palm, inhale, apply to your body, and enjoy the mood boost you'll get from the aromatherapeutic properties of the oil.

POST-COSMETIC SURGERY

If you've had surgery, and you're left with bruises, spider veins, or broken capillaries, a vitamin K cream will make them go away. Massage it in twice a day.

PRODUCTS: Jason Naturals Vitamin K Creme Plus ▪ Reviva Labs Vitamin K Cream ▪ K-Derm Gel.

HORMONAL HEADACHE

Sit in a steam room for five minutes and, in many cases, you'll find that your headache goes away. Create an at-home steam room by turning on the hot water in the shower, leaving the room, and closing the door to the bathroom for a couple of minutes. Go back and inhale for five minutes.

PART III:

the outside world

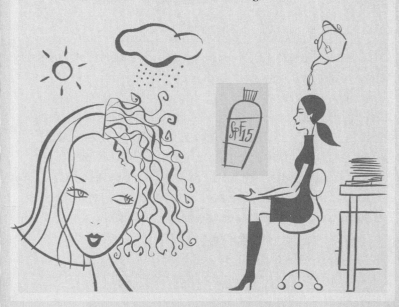

CHAPTER SEVEN

CLIMATE CONTROL

B LAME IT ON THE WEATHER, BUT IT CAN BE HARD to look your best when you're beating back the elements. Saharan summer heat and humidity drive the oil glands crazy and cause breakouts. Winter wind and Arctic chill parch the skin and scalp. Rain and snow can drag down or frizz up your hair. Central heating and air conditioning both generate enough dry air to drive your skin to drink—moisturizer, that is, and lots of it. The seasons can also lift or lower your mood, transform your formerly active self into a couch-crawling cave dweller, and make over your hair and skin in ways you never dreamed possible!

This chapter will offer tips on how to conquer dryness and wind burn, protect against sun damage, strengthen brittle nails, outsmart your oil glands, and triumph over climate in every season.

summer

Summer is the season to kick back, lighten up, and adopt a beauty regimen that's as pared down as your wardrobe. When the weather is warm, most of us prefer less makeup, easy hairstyles, and a smooth, barer body. But summer heat and humidity, the chlorine in the pool, the salt air at the beach, and drying central air conditioning can lead to a multitude of beauty messes.

When summer approaches, it makes good sense to switch to a lighter moisturizer and sheerer makeup, become more vigilant about using sunscreen, exfoliate your face and body regularly, shampoo less often and let your hair air-dry, and keep your pedicure up to date. Here are more ways to cope with summer beauty challenges.

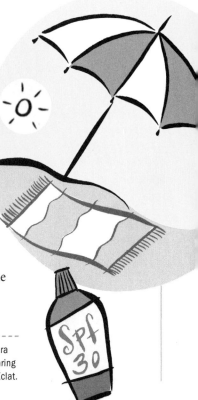

RUNNY CONCEALER

If your concealer tends to run in the summer, try a brush-on pen concealer. These are lightweight, dry quickly, and last.

PRODUCTS: Clinique Airbrush Concealer ■ Laura Mercier Secret Brightener ■ Neutrogena SkinClearing Oil-Free Concealer ■ Yves Saint Laurent Touche Éclat.

SUMMER MAKEUP SWITCHEROO

Certain types of makeup hold up better in the summer heat. Here's your summer checklist:

☐ Oil-free foundation, oil-absorbing makeup, or tinted moisturizer (with SPF 15)

☐ Oil-free powder, blotting paper, or mattifying lotion to absorb oil

☐ Bronzing powder, with undertones of bronze, copper, or gold, to give the face a healthy glow

☐ Powder blush—to help absorb oil—or no blush at all because you'll have natural color

☐ Waterproof mascara—because you'll be sweatier and more active

☐ Lip gloss or lip tint in sheerer shades

MAKEUP MELT

In the sticky summer months, foundation can slide off your face. If you still want some coverage but foundation feels too heavy, switch to a tinted moisturizer (with SPF 15) which offers light, natural-looking coverage with great staying power.

PRODUCTS: L'Occitane Tinted Day Care SPF 15 ■ Dermalogica Sheer Tint Moisture ■ M.D. Formulations Total Protector Color 30 ■ Origins Nude and Improved ■ Stila Sheer Color.

SHINY FACE

With oil glands working overtime in the heat, try mattifying makeup, an amazing makeup technology that soaks up shine and absorbs excess oil like a sponge.

PRODUCTS: Shiseido Pureness Mattifying Stick Oil-Free under your foundation (or without) ■ Chanel Matte Reflecting Makeup ■ Smashbox Anti-Shine ■ Biotherm Sense Matte.

FOIL THE OIL

Trade in your usual moisturizer for a lotion or cream that controls oil production.

PRODUCTS: Lauren Hutton's Good Stuff No Shine Day Cream ■ M·A·C Oil-Control Lotion ■ Aesop Oil-Free Face Hydrating Serum.

T-ZONE TEASE

For an oily T-Zone, blot the face throughout the day with oil-blotting papers—sold at drugstore counters—which will soak up shine right away.

LIPSTICK OVERLOAD

For the sheerest lip color, apply lipstick, tinted lip balm, or gloss with your finger instead of applying it directly from the tube or with a lip brush (a brush will leave a brush stroke on your lips). Press it into your lips until it looks like a soft stain.

TOO-DARK BRONZER

Choose a bronzer in a shade lighter than you think you need, because bronzer turns dark after it mingles with the oils in your skin. For oily skin, use a gel stick or gel in a tube. For dry skin, use a bronzing lotion or cream. Bronzing powder works well on all skin types.

STREAKY BRONZER

To beat streaking apply less than you think you need; you can always add more later. Apply bronzer wherever the sun would naturally hit your face—along the hairline, blended upward along the apples of the cheeks, and along the jawline.

SCALY FEET

Come warm weather, the prospect of exposing your scaly winter feet may be daunting. Apply a moisturizing face mask (yes, a face mask!) to the dry, scaly tops of your feet and toes. Leave on overnight, and when you wake up, your feet will be baby-soft.

PRODUCTS: Eau Thermale Avène Instant Soothing Moisture Mask ■ Boscia Moisture Replenishing Mask.

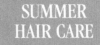

SUMMER HAIR CARE

■ Because you'll probably be shampooing more often, use a gentle, moisturizing shampoo and conditioner.

■ If you've lightened your hair for the summer, switch to a shampoo for color-treated hair.

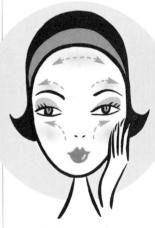

Apply bronzer along the hairline, temples, and cheeks.

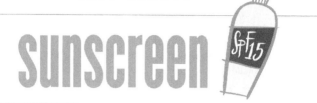

sunscreen

Your most important beauty product

The greatest danger of exposure to ultraviolet radiation is skin cancer. According to the American Cancer Society, more than a million new cases of skin cancer will be diagnosed this year. But skin cancer is almost entirely preventable if you choose the right sunscreen and apply it with slavish devotion. The sun also causes wrinkles, spotty discoloration, and saggy skin, even when you're just out for a quick walk or running an errand in your car (yes, you are exposed in your car).

Make sure that your sunscreen offers broad-spectrum coverage, which will protect you from both UVA and UVB rays. UVA rays cause cancer and premature aging. UVB are the tanning and burning rays. The only way to get protection from both is to apply a sunscreen that lists titanium dioxide, zinc oxide, or Parsol 1789 (avobenzene) as an

Use a sun stick to get at hard to reach spots.

active ingredient. (If you have sensitive skin or rosacea, and sunscreen makes your skin sting, stick with a sunscreen that lists titanium dioxide or zinc oxide as active ingredients, rather than avobenzene, which may irritate sensitive skin.) Look for a minimum SPF of 15, which is high enough, unless you're very fair. A higher SPF is not always better, and here's why.

SPF 15 will shield you from about 94 percent of the sun's rays; an SPF 30 will only increase your protection to 97 percent, and it may increase the risk of skin irritation, especially if you have sensitive skin. But if you are fair and burn easily, that extra 3 percent may make a difference. Always apply sunscreen at least 15 minutes before you head outdoors to give the ingredients time to bond with your skin. And don't forget about the spots that are easy to overlook: behind the ears, on the earlobes, on the eyelids, and under the eyes.

How much sunscreen do you need to apply to your face on a fine summer day? In general, apply the same amount of sunscreen as you would apply lotion to dry skin. And don't forget to reapply. Sunscreen runs off as you sweat and, of course, after you go in the water.

HOW HANDY

Don't forget to protect the skin on the backs of your hands from sun damage. After you apply sunscreen to your face (and neck!) wipe the excess from each palm onto the back of the other hand.

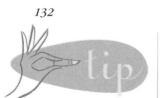

TAN LINES TIP

*Don't give up on
your strapless dress.
Take a barely damp
makeup sponge, dip
it in bronzer, and
cover up those tan
lines. Make sure to
blend very well, and
top with a light
sweep of bronzing
powder.*

SUNSCREEN BREAKOUTS

If your skin is oily or blemish-prone, use a clear liquid or oil-free gel formulation, because it is less likely to clog your pores than greasy lotions or creams. Or, try a spray, because sprays are lighter and less occlusive.

PRODUCTS: Clinique Body Spray SPF 15 Sun Block ▪ Bobbi Brown Sunscreen Body Spray SPF 15 ▪ DDF Sun Gel.

SUNSCREEN IN YOUR EYES

Apply lip balm with SPF 15 around the eyes or use a sun stick. These are thicker, less runny, and more water resistant than regular sunscreens.

PRODUCTS: Dr. Hauschka Skin Care Sun-Block SPF 30 ▪ Clarins Sun Control Stick.

SAKE FOR SUN SPOTS

Fade out sun spots with sake. Kojic acid (a popular skin lightener) was discovered in koji (sake), and in Japan, people rub sake on their skin daily to lighten dark spots. It takes at least four weeks to see results. Or, look for lightening products with kojic acid or licorice extract (glycyrrhizinate).

PRODUCTS: SCO Clarifying Complex ▪ SkinCeuticals Phyto + ▪ Shiseido Whiteners Intensive Skin Brightener ▪ Nuskin Triphasic White ▪ Neostrata Brightening Cream.

SUMMER RUDOLF

It's easy for sunscreen to slide off your nose—it's the oiliest part of your face. If you're as red-nosed as Rudolf after time in

STING RAYS

Sunburn can be painful and cause blisters. Of course, the idea is *never ever* to bake in the sun like a slab of clay in the Arizona desert, but if you fell asleep in the sun or got caught up in a volleyball game, here's what to do.

■ If your burn isn't too bad, slit an aloe leaf and apply it to the skin to relieve stinging and redness. But if you need to soothe vast swaths of your sunburned skin, break open a few aloe leaves and float them in a cool bath. Soak for ten minutes.

■ Dump half a jar of Nestea in a bath, and soak.

■ Steep two regular tea bags in boiling water. Let cool. Pat the bags on your face for five to ten minutes. The tannic acid draws out the burn. (This will soothe any burn, not just sunburn.)

■ Take Advil or another over-the-counter anti-inflammatory every four hours

to reduce redness and soothe the swelling.

■ Apply an antioxidant cream—with green or white tea, vitamin E, or shea butter—or lavender oil, which can reduce the redness and neutralize free-radical damage.

■ Drink lots of water—you're likely to be dehydrated, and it will make you feel better.

■ To prevent blisters: Apply a compress soaked in red wine vinegar and ice to sun-baked skin.

■ To soothe peeling skin: Dip a cloth in a mix of half cool water, half apple

SUNSTROKE IS NOT TO BE TAKEN LIGHTLY. If you have any of these symptoms—dizziness, chills, nausea, difficulty breathing —call your doctor.

cider vinegar, and pat it on bits of peeling skin on chest or shoulders. Apply moisturizing body oil. Certain oils (buckthorn, sweet almond, sesame) not only act as intense moisturizers, they absorb more quickly into the skin, and you'll see faster results.

- - - - - - - - - - - -
PRODUCTS: Weleda Sea Buckthorn Body Oil ■ Sweet almond oil (found in health-food stores) ■ Neutrogena Sesame Body Oil ■ Dr. Hauschka Skin Care After-Sun Lotion ■ Kneipp Spa Massage Oil.

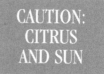

CAUTION: CITRUS AND SUN

Lemon (or lime) juice will keep bugs away, and it will also highlight your hair. But on the skin, citric acid reacts to the sun and causes brown spots called berloque dermatitis. (Citrus-based perfume can cause the same reaction, which is why it's not a good idea to wear it in the sun.) The spots will eventually go away, but in the meantime, cover them up with makeup *and* sunscreen, because repeated sun exposure can make them permanent.

the sun, cover your nose with a creamy beige concealer until the red starts to fade. Steer clear of pink- or green-toned concealer. Next time, set your sunscreen with a little translucent powder, and it will hold better. And reapply sunscreen to your nose.

SUNSCREEN PALLOR

Your sunscreen gives your skin a whitish cast. Mix a dollop of foundation or tinted moisturizer in your palm with your sunscreen before you apply to your skin.

SELF-TANNER SELF-STARTER

First, exfoliate, then mix a small dab of self-tanner with a squirt of moisturizer, and apply it to your pasty limbs. The moisturizer will smooth out dry patches so the tanner doesn't streak.

PRODUCTS: Clarins Self Tanning Milk or Self Tanning Instant Gel ■ Sothys Self-Tanner Illuminating Express.

SELF-TANNER FADE-OUT

When your self-tan has that leftover look, use a face or body scrub to even out your skin tone.

PRODUCTS: Laura Mercier Face Polish ■ Avalon Organic Botanicals Exfoliating Enzyme Scrub ■ Astara Daily Refining Scrub.

SELF-TANNER SPLOTCHES

Before you apply your self-tanner, dab a bit of body lotion on spots where it tends to collect and get too dark, like your ankles, knees, and toes. To erase a streaky mistake, try St. Tropez Self-Tan Remover.

FAKE A GOLDEN GLEAM

Apply a shimmery body lotion to give your skin—especially shoulders and legs—a golden gleam.

PRODUCTS: Nivea Silky Shimmer Lotion ■ Prescriptives Sunsheen Body Tint ■ Jergens Natural Glow Daily Moisturizer.

SWEATY FEET

Sweaty feet can be a problem, especially when they're trapped in synthetic shoes or plastic sandals. Wear natural-fiber socks, go barefoot, or wear open-toe sandals to let your feet breathe. Soak feet in cool water spiked with apple cider vinegar or chilled tea, which decreases perspiration.

SANDAL-WORTHY

At the Sweet Lily Natural Nail Spa in New York City, owner Donna Perillo sweetens the feet with all-natural ingredients. Here's her recipe for whipping your dogs into sandal-ready shape: Grind ½ cup each of walnuts and brown sugar and 2 teaspoons each of honey, almond oil, and jojoba oil in a food processor. Massage into damp feet. Rinse, and follow with moisturizer.

HARD HEELS

Use a body scrub on your heels in the shower, then run a pumice stone over

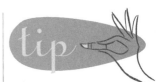

SELF-TANNER STAINS

After applying self-tanner, always wash your hands immediately. But if your hands do stain, rub half a lemon on them, then moisturize. Or, massage a body scrub into your hands, repeatedly, over the course of a few hours.

SORE, TIGHT APRES-SUN SKIN

Apply plain yogurt to the skin, leave on for ten minutes, and rinse with cool water. Use whatever yogurt you have—whole-milk, low-fat, or fat-free.

them. Before you go to bed, apply a rich glycolic acid cream, and cover with socks. Leave on overnight.

PRODUCTS: Eucerin Plus Intensive Repair Lotion ▪ Glytone Ultra Heel and Elbow Cream ▪ Clinique Water Therapy Foot Smoothing Cream ▪ Origins Reinventing the Heel ▪ MD Formulations Pedicreme.

DISAPPEARING ACT

To keep your fragrance from evaporating quickly in the hot summer months, squirt a dab of fragrance-free moisturizer in your palm, mix in a few drops of your fragrance, and massage it into your skin.

ODOR-FREE PRODUCTS: Osea Ocean Lotion ▪ Origins Constant Comforter.

INFECTED BIKINI BUMPS

Apply acne medicine or antibiotic ointment like Neosporin at night. To cover them up at the beach, apply waterproof makeup or concealer with salicylic acid.

PRODUCTS: Clinique Acne Solutions Concealing Cream ▪ Neutrogena SkinClearing Oil-Free Concealer.

BIKINI LINE STING

Because waxing can make skin sun-sensitive, wax a couple of days before you head off on your beach vacation. If your bikini line begins to sting, soothe it with aloe vera gel. Shower after going in salt water and don't expose to the sun.

PRODUCTS: Brave Soldier Code Blue ▪ Clinique CX Rapid Recovery Cream ▪ Aquaphor Healing Ointment.

COLD SORES

Cold sores are often aggravated by exposure to UV light, which is why they're most common during the summer. They can also be triggered by lip waxing, laser treatments, peels, Retin-A, and stress. Dab on Pepto-Bismol as soon as you feel one. If they recur often, ask your doctor to prescribe Famvir, Valtrex, or Zovirax, and use it *as soon as you feel a cold sore coming.*

SUPER-SENSITIVE SKIN

Glycolic acids make the skin extra-sensitive to waxing, especially during the summer. If you use glycolics regularly on your face, tweeze your brows instead of waxing them.

NAIL POLISH TURNS YELLOW

Many nail polish brands contain the adhesive nitrocellulose, which can turn yellow when exposed to sunlight. Apply a topcoat that contains cellulose acetate butyrate (CAB) over your nail polish, and it will prevent your nails from discoloration.

PRODUCTS: Seche Vite Dry Fast Top Coat ▪ Orly Sunscreen for Nails ▪ Essie Nonyellowing Topcoat.

FUNKY NAIL COLOR

If gardening or other outdoor work causes your nails to discolor, apply Crest whitening strips to your nails—it works as well as it does on your teeth.

What can I do about bikini bumps and ingrown hairs?

If you have curly or wavy hair, you're especially prone. To keep your bikini line smooth, exfoliate with a body scrub every time you shower. Follow up after you wax or shave with a product that has salicylic acid, beta hydroxy acid, tea tree oil, or antioxidants to soothe the skin and keep the bumps at bay.

PRODUCTS: Oloff Beauty Rash Decision ▪ Bliss Ingrown Hair Eliminating Peeling Pads ▪ Terax Original Body Pr' Ax ▪ Bikini Blaster Pads ▪ Tendskin ▪ Astara AHA Nutrient Toning Essence.

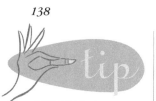

SUMMER SHIMMER

Apply a solid-color polish, and layer a shimmer polish on top. The shimmer keeps the color correct and looks great in the sun.

STAINED NAILS

To remove stains on your nails, soak them in juice of one lemon diluted in 1 cup water. Or, dip a sponge, loofah, or other abrasive in white wine vinegar and scrub. Or, use a body scrub on your nails.

NAILS WON'T DRY

A dip in a bowl of water with ice will quick-dry polish that takes forever in sticky weather.

MOISTURIZER MELTDOWN

In hot weather, stash your gel, lotion, or cream—especially eye cream—in the fridge. The chill feels good on your skin, keeps the product from breaking down in the heat, and helps tone your skin, too.

FADED COLOR

If your hair color has faded, perk it up with a color-depositing or color-enhancing shampoo every other wash, until the color deepens. (Don't use it every day, or it will weigh down your hair.)

PRODUCTS: Aura Clove Shampoo (brunettes), Madder Root Shampoo (redheads), or Blue Malva Shampoo (blondes) ■ Mine Shampoo ■ Te Tao Colour Enhancing Shampoo.

TURNING GREEN

If chlorine tends to turn your bottle-blond hair green, (1) rinse your hair with seltzer or club soda as soon as you come out of the pool; (2) rinse with tomato juice or massage

PROTECT YOUR HAIR COLOR

Sun, surf, chlorine, and salt air can fade your hair color, fast! The sun reacts with chemically treated hair to oxidize the color, and the only way to retard it is to cover up with a hat or scarf. Sunscreens for the hair don't really work. Here's some other advice to "set" your hair color and keep it from fading:

▓ Wait at least 24 to 48 hours after you color your hair before washing it.

▓ Comb a protective conditioner through wet or dry hair before you swim.

▓ Wash or rinse your hair as soon as possible after swimming.

▓ Use a gentle shampoo that targets color-treated hair.

▓ Don't shampoo your hair every day.

Water oxidizes color even more than sun and makes it fade faster.

▓ Don't overdry your hair. If you use a blow-dryer, keep the temperature on low.

ketchup through your hair to get rid of the green. (See Chapter 10, page 202.)

SUMMER STATIC

Humidity can create flyaways in straight hair. After you moisturize, run your palms over your dry hair. The leftover moisturizer will smooth the flyaways. Or spray a nonaerosol hair spray on your hairbrush, and brush through your hair (aerosol spray is too light to work).

A TANGLED MESS

Sun exposure can rough up hair strands and cause them to tangle. Before you swim, slick a bit of leave-in conditioner through dry or damp hair.

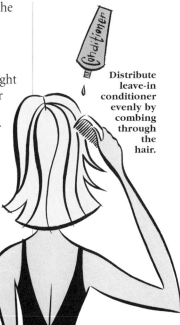

Distribute leave-in conditioner evenly by combing through the hair.

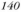
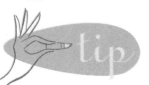

SALTWATER SEXY

Remember how thick and sexy your hair looks after a day at the beach? It's the salt, silly. So if your hair flattens around 4 P.M., spray it with saltwater and give it a tousle. The water will reactivate the products in your hair, and the salt will thicken it.

PRODUCTS: Lavett & Chin Seasalt Thickening Mist ■ Lush Big Shampoo.

DRY HAIR

L ook for hydrating treatments and masks with ingredients that end in *-amine,* for amino acids that strengthen hair.

PRODUCTS: Pantene Deep Hydrating Treatment (all hair types) ■ John Frieda FrizzEase Miraculous Recovery Deep Conditioning Treatment (curly hair) ■ Lancôme Force Densite Extra Density Replenishing Mask (fine hair).

STRAIGHT FRIZZ

E ven straight hair can get frizzy. To beat back the frizz, mix a dime-size dab of gel in your palm with a dab of pomade and pat through your hair. Apply a mix of leave-in conditioner and gel to wet hair.

PRODUCTS: Tressa Texturizing Paste (for short, spiky styles) ■ Hairgum Pomade (vegetable pomade).

CURLY FRIZZ

R ub a bit of shine serum between your palms and pat throughout your hair. It will keep it from frizzing and add shine. Or, put a dab of hairstyling cream in your palms, and scrunch it through your hair.

ALL FRIZZY HAIR

S pray with a nonaerosol hairspray, which will give your hair hold, beat back the frizz, and leave it feeling touchable, too.

SOFTER CURLS

I f your hair is curly and you want to define your curls, rub a bit of hair cream between your palms, wrap a piece of hair (¼ inch for tight curls, ½ inch for looser curls) around your index finger, and release. Continue around your entire head. Let your hair dry naturally or blow-dry on a low setting with a diffuser.

HAIR LIFT

To give your hairstyle a quick lift, apply gel to a few hair clips, clip them into the front of your hair, lifting the hair slightly, and leave in for ten minutes. Or, turn your head upside down, spray volumizer into the roots, and scrunch, starting at the roots.

PRODUCTS: Aveda Volumizing Tonic ▪ Nexxus Vita Tress Conditioning Volumizer ▪ Frédéric Fekkai Instant Volume Spray.

SUN-SCORCHED HAIR

Apply a leave-in conditioner or conditioning mask.

PRODUCTS: Pantene Pro-V Overnight Repair Intensive Treatment ▪ Kerastase Nutri-Liss ▪ L'Oréal Vive Smooth-Intense Masque (for frizzy hair) ▪ Warren-Tricomi Cabana Collection Leave-In Conditioner.

HOT HEAD

If you must blow-dry your hair in summer, first blot it dry with a towel really well to minimize dryer time. Then, only blow-dry around the hairline. Keep your dryer on the cool or medium setting throughout the summer to reduce dryness. Think about investing in an ionic dryer, which cuts drying time in half and neutralizes the hair's electrostatic charge, which means less frizz.

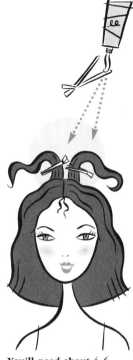

You'll need about 4–6 clips to "lift" the top of your hairstyle.

winter

Cold weather seems to sap every drop of moisture from the skin and hair. Even the nails become brittle when the temperature drops and drier air moves in. Whether it's caused by a warm woolen cap (hat hair), a cozy fireplace (flushed face), a day on the ski slopes (windburn), or a simple walk outdoors (all of the above), the result is a beauty distress call: dry hair, dandruff, cracked nails, flaky skin, "alligator claws," and worse. When the weather is at its most harsh, your beauty regimen should be at its most gentle. Here's your winter regime change.

Switch to a cream-based cleanser, along with a thicker moisturizer or emollient oil. To counteract dry, flaky skin, gently exfoliate so that the skin can absorb moisturizer better. Unless your skin is extremely oily, cut back your cleansing routine by rinsing with just water in the morning, and save the cleanser for bedtime. Too much cleansing strips the skin of "natural" protective oils. Don't forget to use a hand cream, and pamper your hair with a deep-conditioning treatment every few weeks.

WINTER: THE SEASONAL SWITCHEROO

Certain types of makeup—and haircare techniques—are better suited for cold weather. Here's your winter checklist:

WINTER MAKEUP

☐ Creamy or "luminous" (light-reflecting) foundation to counter dryness and give the skin a glow with undertones of peach, apricot and pink to warm up washed-out, wan-looking skin

☐ Pressed or translucent powder

☐ Cream blush

☐ Creamy lipstick

☐ Nonwaterproof mascara (waterproof can be drying)

WINTER HAIR

☐ Shampoo less frequently—twice a week, unless your hair is oily.

☐ Avoid the high setting on your blow-dryer, and, whenever possible, let your hair dry naturally.

PALE FACE

Warm your skin with a touch of bronzing gel mixed with moisturizer. Or, lighten the hair around your face, which brightens up the skin.

CHAPPED LIPS

Gently exfoliate lips with a toothbrush and Vaseline, your face scrub, or an exfoliating lip product. Then apply lip balm.

PRODUCTS: Clinique All About Lips ▪ Benefit Cosmetics Lipscription.

Use a soft-bristle toothbrush to exfoliate your lips.

WINTER BLUES

Think pink or peach cream blush or cheek gel, which warms up any skin, even in the dead of winter. If your skin is medium to dark, try a deeper apricot.

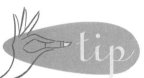

ITCHY SNAKE SKIN

Wrap a handful of oatmeal in a washcloth or cheesecloth and run it under hot water until soaked. Sit on the edge of the tub and rest the oat poultice on dry, itchy areas, squeezing gently for a few minutes. Or soak in a warm— not hot—oatmeal bath. Then, spray skin with Aveeno Anti-Itch Gel Spray or Soothing Care Itch Relief Spray.

DRY LIPS

Products with camphor, like Blistex or Carmex, can dry the lips. Look for lip balm with shea butter or beeswax.

PRODUCTS: Burt's Bees Beeswax Lip Balm ■ L'Occitane Shea Butter Lip Balm ■ Jurlique Lip Care Balm ■ Eau Thermale Avène Lip Balm with Cold Cream.

DRY SKIN, TIGHT FACE

Mist your face with cool water and pat dry before you apply moisturizer. It will plump up your skin, pronto.

SUPER DRY SKIN

After a bath or shower, pat your skin with a towel, but leave it damp. Then, massage moisturizer into your skin for a couple of minutes—don't just pat and run—so that it has time to absorb. (Keep the bathroom door closed after your bath or shower, to trap steam while you apply cream.)

WHEN A TINGLE BECOMES A CHILL

A chilly bathroom can chill your face and your moisturizer. Put a dab of cream (or lotion) into your palm, cup your other hand on top for a minute or two to warm it, then apply. It will feel better and will absorb better into the skin as well.

RUDOLF NOSE

Before you head outdoors on a windy day (or when your nose is irritated from a cold), dip a Q-tip in Vaseline and apply a tiny bit to the lower rim of your nostrils to prevent a sore, red, chapped nose.

COLD SHOULDER

To warm up pallid skin revealed in a strappy little evening dress, apply a dab of body oil to shoulders, back, chest, and décolleté, then brush on shimmer powder with a big powder brush. Your skin will glow!

NOT-SO-SWEET FEET

Your feet have more than 250,000 sweat glands, and when they're trapped inside your boots all day, sweat happens. Rotate your shoes and boots so you give them a day to dry out and air beween wearings. For day, massage baking soda, arrowroot powder, or cornstarch into your feet. These products work as well on your feet as they do on refrigerator odors. And try a foot deodorizer, or place odor-absorbing insoles in your boots.

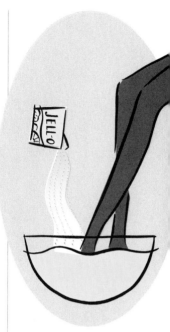

At night, soak sweaty feet in a bowl of Jell-O. It works!

PRODUCTS: Gold Bond Foot Spray ▪ Gold Bond Foot Powder ▪ Dr. Scholl's Odor Destroyers Shoe Freshener Women's Insoles.

LIP CRACKS

In cold, windy weather, you may develop little cracks around the corners of your mouth, that are often caused by yeast infections. Massage a dab of Lamisil or Lotrimin, both antifungal creams, into the cracks, being careful to keep it out of the mouth. While they heal, which takes about a week, try to avoid lipstick and apply Vaseline instead.

RUDDY SKIN

If you're naturally fair, your face may turn ruddy and irritated from the wind and cold. Apply a cool cloth to your cheeks after you come inside. It prevents your blood vessels from dilating as a response to the radical temperature change. And try these anti-inflammatory products, which will take down the irritation.

PRODUCTS: Prescriptives Redness Relief Gel ■ Clinique CX Redness Relief Cream ■ NuSkin Epoch Calming Touch Soothing Skin Cream ■ Eucerin Redness Relief Daily Perfecting Lotion.

When you exfoliate with a natural bristle brush, always brush toward the heart.

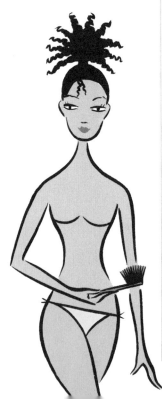

ASHY SKIN

In winter, African-American women can be especially prone to "ash"—a pale, dusty buildup of dry skin all over the body. To restore your skin's glow, brush with a natural-bristle brush on dry skin before you enter the shower, and moisturize with a lotion that contains glycerin, which attracts moisture to the skin.

PRODUCTS: Jergens Ash Relief Moisturizer ■ Olay Quench Body Lotion ■ L'Occitane Body Balm Honey Harvest.

BABY BUMPS

Those small bumps on the backs of your arms and legs are caused when dead skin piles up around a hair follicle. They're especially common when your body is bundled in heavy layers all winter. Exfoliate every time you bathe or shower, with a sponge, loofah, body scrub, or buff puff. After showering, apply moisturizer, and the bumps should disappear within two weeks.

PRODUCTS: Neutrogena Skin Smoothing Body Lotion ▪ MD Formulations Glycolic Hand and Body Cream ▪ Eucerin Plus Intensive Repair Lotion.

SLOW-GRO NAILS

Winter slows everything down, even nail growth. To make your nails grow faster during the slow-gro season, take omega-3 (fish oil) supplements (which are found in any health-food store).

THE NAIL-CHIP NIPPER

To extend the life of your manicure, use a topcoat along with this trick: After each coat of polish, bring the brush along the edge of the nail. After you apply the topcoat, bring the brush under the tip of each nail for extra protection that will nip that chip before it happens.

ONION-PEEL NAILS

To strengthen dry, peeling nails, soak your hands in warm milk. Pat dry. Then, moisturize your nails with a good nail strengthener.

PRODUCTS: Essie Millionails Nail Strengthener ▪ DDF Anti-Fungal Cuticle and Nail Treatment ▪ Dr. Hauschka Neem Nail Oil.

SCALY HANDS

Keep your body scrub by the bathroom sink. After you wash your hands, massage with scrub.

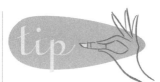

COLD HANDS

Try a hand cream with mint, rosemary, or ginger, which stimulates circulation and brings warmth to the area, or tuck a Japanese-style hand warmer into your gloves or purse.

THE JOB AT HAND

In the 1800s, European women slept with moisturizing gloves brushed inside with rose water, almond oil, and egg yolk. Some even wrapped their hands in raw meat to "tenderize" them overnight. These days, a good hand cream will do the job. Look for a lotion or cream with glycerin and plant oils, which absorb well into the skin and leave no tacky residue. Apply hand cream at least twice a day, especially after washing your hands.

PRODUCTS: Jurlique Lavender or Rose Hand Cream ▪ Ole Henriksen Hands Forward Cream ▪ Eau Thermale Avène Hand Cream with Cold Cream ▪ Kiehl's Ultimate Strength Hand Salve ▪ Neutrogena Norwegian Formula Hand Cream.

ALLIGATOR CLAWS

Dry, chapped hands are more prone to infection, because bacteria can more easily sneak into cracks in the skin. Slather your hands and nails with hand cream, slip them into plastic bags, and wrap them in a heating pad for 15 minutes.

PRODUCTS: Elizabeth Arden Eight-Hour Cream Intensive Moisturizer Hand Treatment ▪ Nivea Restorative Night Hand Creme ▪ Sally Hansen 18-Hour Protective Hand Creme.

HEAVY-DUTY FLAKES

Cut the toes off stretchy cotton sports socks, apply a heavy moisturizer on elbows and knees, and pull the socks over them before you go to bed.

PRODUCTS: Palmer's Shea Butter Formula Lotion ▪ Kiehls Intensive Treatment and Moisturizer ▪ St. Ives 24-Hour Moisture.

FLAKY KNEES AND ELBOWS

Exfoliate dry skin with a natural-bristle brush or an old toothbrush. Warm a bit of olive or sweet almond oil, pour it in two little bowls, and soak your elbows in them for ten minutes. Wipe dry, then moisturize with a rich cream.

FAST FLAKE BUSTER

To soften knees and elbows in a flash, roll on a bit of "emollient to go."

PRODUCTS: Fresh Sugar Shea Butter To Go ▪ Nature's Gate Organics Body Stick.

FLAKY PATCH

To shed a flaky patch of skin on your face, look for creams with lactic acid, a type of alpha hydroxy acid.

PRODUCTS: AmLactin XL Moisturizing Lotion ■ Neutrogena Healthy Skin Face Lotion.

SLO-GLO

If your legs are too pale even for the winter, try Jergens Daily Glow, a body lotion pre-mixed with tanner.

WIND-WHIPPED

Before you head out to the slopes, apply a thick cream with occlusive ingredients like dimethicone or shea butter to shield and soothe your skin from windchill and wind-burn.

PRODUCTS: Kiehl's All-Sport "Non-Freeze" Face Protector SPF 30 ■ Clinique Moisture Surge Extra Thirsty Skin Relief ■ Dermalogica Barrier Repair.

HOT HEAD

Protect hair from hot blow-dryer blasts with heat-protection products.

PRODUCTS: Paul Mitchell Heat Seal ■ Redken Spray Starch ■ Pantene Heat Protector Spray.

ITCHY SCALP

Cold air that constricts the veins can leave your scalp feeling tight and itchy. Before shampooing, brush your scalp gently with a natural-bristle brush to stimulate the circulation and ease the itch. Plus, it feels good!

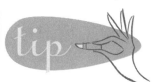

GO FOR THE GLOW

Wet a washcloth with warm water and squeeze the juice of a lime on the cloth. Press onto your face, and leave on for a few minutes. Repeat two or three times. You'll glow like you've just stood on your head in yoga class.

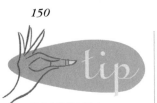

MASCARA MOMENT

When the wind is blowing, your eyes are tearing, and your mascara's running, you'll wish you'd tried this: After applying a coat of mascara, dip a Q-tip into loose powder and tip on your wet lashes. Then apply a second coat of mascara.

DRY SCALP

Before you shampoo your hair, rinse your hair and scalp with apple cider. It will soothe a tight, dry scalp and remove any excess buildup from your styling products.

FRINGE BENEFITS

French women use lash extenders that go on with a mascara wand. While lashes are still wet from putting on one coat of mascara, apply Longcil Extender, which has little fibers that stick to the mascara. Apply a second coat of mascara and—voila!

DULL HAIR

Spray a bit of camellia oil or a light kitchen oil on your palms, rub them together, and pat on your hair.

PRODUCTS: Darphin Protective Shining Oil with Camellia ■ Leonor Greyl Magnolia Oil.

BONE-DRY HAIR

Don't shampoo. Just apply conditioner to wet or dry hair. Cover with a plastic cap, and busy yourself around the house for ten to 15 minutes. The heat of your body trapped under the plastic cap warms the conditioner so it penetrates better. Rinse, and see how soft and shiny your hair looks!

BRITTLE HAIR

Apply your normal conditioner to wet or dry hair. Dampen a towel and put it in the microwave for 20 seconds. Wrap around your hair and leave on for 15 minutes.

BLOWING IN THE WIND

If you live in a windy city but don't like the windblown look, apply leave-in conditioner before you leave the house, and pull your hair back in a loose ponytail. When you get to the office, give your hair a gentle shake.

HAT HAIR

If your hair needs a lift when you take off your hat, turn your head upside down, shake it, sprinkle a few drops of water on your fingers, and run them through your hair, lifting fingers up in a jagged motion. The water will reactivate your styling products and give your hair a lift.

ALL WORKED UP

If you wake up with your hair standing on end, try sleeping on a satin pillowcase. Satin won't cause friction, which can work up your hair. When you comb your hair, don't start at the roots, but at the ends, then inch your way up.

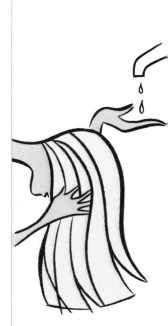

Turn your head upside down and shake some air into your hair.

FADEOUT

Natural hair color fades too, especially from too much sun and too many winter-warm-up hot showers. Wash hair in cool water, try a color-brightening shampoo (look for "non-color" deposit), and apply hair gel with shimmer particles to perk things up in the meantime.

Transitional Seasons:
Spring and Fall

When the seasons change, your skin may need some special therapy to ease the transition. To see if your skin is dehydrated, gently push your cheek up from the jawbone to the cheekbone. If you see lots of tiny lines, it's a distress call.

Replenish the moisture your skin has lost from the drying effects of sun, surf and chlorine. Apply moisturizer and use a small, natural-bristle brush to massage it into the skin. It will

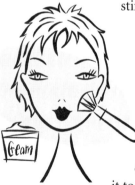

stimulate the circulation and help the moisturizer absorb most effectively. Your skin will immediately look better.

Always try to get a facial between seasons. After the summer, a facial helps to clean out clogged pores, get rid of flaky skin, and clear the skin so that moisturizer penetrates deeper in winter. After winter, a facial helps to clear the dead skin away. If you can't make it to a pro, take 20 minutes on a weekend morning to give yourself an exfoliating and moisturizing mini-facial at home—cleanse, exfoliate, and apply a moisturizing mask to your skin for 15 minutes while puttering around the house.

As Goldilocks might say, autumn is "just right," which is why it tends to balance out or normalize excessively dry or oily hair and skin. Moving from fall to winter, protect your skin by switching to a thicker, more occlusive moisturizer, closer to the consis-

SPRING SHOWERS

Dandruff becomes an even bigger problem in spring and fall. Vinegar can kill the bacteria thought to cause dandruff. Massage a palmful of vinegar onto your clean scalp. Leave it on for two minutes, then rinse. Repeat every day for a week or until you see an improvement. Or try Nizoral, a gentle drugstore dandruff shampoo, or a tea tree oil shampoo.

Dandruff affects African American women 15 to 20 percent more than the general population, according to Dr. Jeanine Downie, author of *Beautiful Skin of Color*. "African American hair is dryer, so it's shampooed less," she says. "And we use a lot of heavy pomades and gels, which build up on the scalp." The way to beat the flakes is to scrub your scalp really well with your fingertips—not your nails—and leave your shampoo on for five minutes.

tency of night cream. From spring to summer, a lighter lotion will do. And throughout every season, *always wear sun protection*.

When your skin color is in transition between seasons, blend your summer and winter foundation together until you hit on the right shade. Or, to stretch that great bronzy glow of summer, use a tinted moisturizer that's a half-shade darker than your skin.

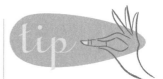

LASH ALERT

To keep your lashes from becoming brittle, gently dab a bit of eye cream on lashes before bed to keep them soft and supple.

CHAPTER EIGHT

STress anD MeDicaTions

OST WOMEN JUGGLE LIVES THAT ARE SO HECTIC, they have little time left over for beauty, let alone anything else. Living a speeded-up lifestyle—always running late, spreading yourself too thin—leads to *stress,* big time! No matter what the source—financial worries, work pressures, multitasking—all stress eventually becomes physical.

The body's response to stress is to release adrenaline, which gives an initial surge of energy, but when stress becomes a daily habit, stress hormones build up in the body. They'll make you feel on edge and burned out—and you'll look that way, too. Common medications that we take to relieve stress can sometimes compound the problem with unexpected beauty-related side effects. When life is this stressful, even the thought of taking time out to relieve it can feel, well, stressful.

At the Golden Door Spa in Escondido, California, a behavioral therapist named Cindi Peterson teaches stressed-out spa-goers about a Japanese philosophy called "kaizen." Loosely translated, *kaizen* means "small baby steps of change," which Peterson is suggesting as a way to break down and manage stress. Taking time out for a relaxing resort or spa vacation may be out of the question, but the idea of kaizen—a small change—"somehow feels manageable, even playful, and it really helps," says Peterson. If you take your stress-busting breaks in bite-sized pieces—a five-minute meditation, a yoga pose, even a restorative face mask—you can manage your stress more easily. You'll be more effective and more productive; you'll feel better and look better, too.

This chapter offers some baby-step suggestions to manage and prevent stress as well as ways to fix the fallout on your body at work and at home. It also has some surprising news about the beauty side effects of many common medications and what to do about them.

Make sure to put stress-relief ideas and "time-outs" on your "to-do" list.

Daily Stress

Too much stress can cause no end of beauty fall-out! Your face may erupt in blemishes, your skin may turn splotchy. Your neck and shoulders will tighten so you hunch when you walk; your nails are bitten to little nubs. Sleep deprivation seems to have left permanent dark circles under your eyes, and your scalp is so dry, you're scratching like a chimp. Here's how to find relief.

SNIFFING COMFORT

In 460 B.C., Hippocrates prescribed fragrance to treat "nervous disorders," the quaint, old-fashioned term for stress. It's no secret that good smells make you feel better, and studies at the Smell and Taste Treatment and Research Foundation have proven it. Instead of whipping up a batch of chocolate-chip cookies and eating half the dough, open a bottle of vanilla extract and take a quick sniff.

ALL WRUNG OUT

To recharge your batteries when your energy is low, do what great bathing cultures of the world have done for centuries: Take a hot-cold plunge. Start with a warm shower. Increase the temperature to really warm, then switch to a burst of cold, then back to really warm. Don't overdo it, however; a cycle of one to four rotations is enough. *If you are pregnant or have high blood pressure, don't try this.*

HEAD AND NECK TENSION

Massage your scalp with your fingertips in small, circular motions to release tension and your skin will glow.

IRRITATED SKIN

French women use thermal water on their skin—with selenium, an anti-inflammatory—and we should, too.

PRODUCTS: Vichy Laboratories Thermal Lotion ▪ La Roche Posay Rosaliac Skin Perfecting Anti-Redness Thermal Spray.

LOW ENERGY FLOW

Dry-brush your body before you step into the shower in the morning. With a long-handled natural-bristle brush or loofah (from the health-food store or the bath and body shop), brush your legs, then arms, from the tips of your fingers and toes toward the heart. Brush your torso toward the heart, as well, but be gentle with the breast area, and avoid the face. Your body will tingle slightly, from your revved-up circulation, and you'll feel that old get-up-and-go!

FEELING JUMPY?

Run your wrists under cold water for a couple of minutes to calm yourself down.

TIED IN KNOTS

Even lobsters relax when given a little massage—their eye stalks go limp! When you can't reach the tight spots on your upper back and shoulders, lie on your back on the floor and roll on top of a rolling pin or a tennis ball until you've untangled the knots.

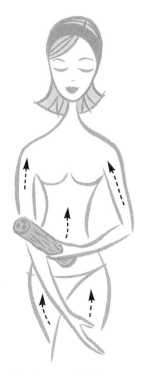

Two-for-one: Exfoliate your skin and stimulate your circulation.

BIG ZIT'S A COMIN'

There's nothing like stress to bring on a pimple. If you feel one on the way before you go to bed, apply a site-specific salicylic acid medication, and, if you're lucky, the pimple will be gone by bugle call.

PRODUCTS: Clean & Clear Overnight Acne Patches ▪ Bye Bye Blemish Drying Lotion ▪ Neutrogena On-the-Spot Acne Patch.

stress makes a mess

Pimple Remedies

Pimples when you're 30? 35? Adult acne can come as a shock, especially when you thought you'd finally outgrown the trials of adolescence. Well, nothing churns up those sneaky little sebaceous glands like stress. For teens, most acne is localized around the T-Zone, while adult acne clusters around the mouth and chin. Here are the most common treatments for minor breakouts. Some require a prescription, others don't. Most mild acne can be kept under check with a consistent cleansing regimen, including spot medication, and an occasional facial (every six weeks). If you've got a severe case of acne, visit a dermatologist. (See Beauty Meltdowns, pages 48–49, and Tweens and Teens, pages 63–67 for more on blemishes.)

■ **Salicylic acid** cleansers and over-the-counter spot treatments unclog pores to heal pimples.

■ **Tea tree oil** kills bacteria that cause acne and dries up pimples.

■ **Glycolic acid creams** or chemical peels exfoliate the top layer of skin to remove dead skin cells and excess sebum and loosen blackheads.

■ **Retinoids** (vitamin A derivatives) like Differin, Tazorac, tretinoin, and Avita normalize the shedding of skin cells, but can cause dryness, redness, and flakiness. *Can be risky for pregnant women.*

■ **Topical antibiotics** like clindamycin (Cleocin) and sulfonamide (Klaron) kill bacteria.

BRAIN DRAIN

Lie across your bed and hang your head over the edge. You'll get your blood rushing to your brain (where it should be, anyway!), which will stimulate circulation to your skin cells, so that you'll look and feel more awake.

STRESS BITES

To keep me from biting my nails my mother used to tell me to sit on my hands, which was a problem, because I seem to need my hands to talk! Instead, keep a tube of hand cream in your purse. When you want to bite your nails, apply it, and the taste will act as a deterrent. Like one of Pavlov's dogs, you'll eventually condition yourself not to bite.

RAGGEDY CUTICLES

If you have really dry cuticles, which makes them more tempting to bite—don't! Rub them with olive oil (olive contains squalene, a great moisturizer) or cuticle cream.

PRODUCTS: Kiehl's Imperiale Moisturizing Cuticle Treatment ▪ Nailtiques Cuticle and Hand Conditioner ▪ Aquaphor Healing Ointment ▪ MD Formulations Nail and Cuticle Complex.

CALM THE SAVAGE BEAST

As part of your party primping, relax in a tub sprinkled with aromatherapy bath oils, as the ancient Greeks did. "Here she bathes," said Homer, "and round her body pours soft oils of fragrance and ambrosial

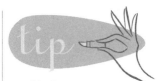

CUTICLE CRISIS

No cuticle cream? Grab your lip balm and massage it into your cuticles to soften them and help keep the temptation to bite at bay.

MONKEY MIND

In Buddhism they say you need to rid yourself of "monkey mind"—a Buddhist phrase that means your thoughts are scattered—to empty your mind for relaxation and stress relief.

showers." Massage relaxing bath oil all over your body *before* you step into the bath. The oil will disperse into the water, the scent will relax you, and your skin will feel soft and silky.

NERVOUS NELLIE

Practice a minute or two of alternate nostril breathing to calm yourself down. Take a deep breath in through the nose, put your thumb over your right nostril, breathe out through your left. Breathe in through your left nostril, then put your index finger over your left nostril and breathe out through the right. Continue this way, exhaling and inhaling on one side, then switch nostrils.

NEED A LITTLE ZEST?

A whiff of orange helps lift the spirits and calm the nerves in the form of oils (neroli), perfumes, lotions, potpourri, and, of course, the real thing—eat an orange.

PRODUCTS: Comptoir Sud Pacifique Coeur de Vahine ■ Aesop Rind Aromatique Body Balm.

HEADACHE HELL

Studies have shown that the cause of most migraines can be directly linked to a magnesium and calcium deficiency in the body. Make sure to get your RDA dose of these minerals, and see if your migraines migrate. Avoid triggers like red wine, cheese, caffeine, and chocolate.

GOT A HUNCH?

Have you ever seen a woman who hunches up her "bag" shoulder, even when she's not carrying a bag? The body holds stress—physical and emotional—in strange ways, which is why it's so important to be aware of your posture. Look at the way you stand in the mirror. If you're hunching, drop your shoulders down. Circle your shoulders back several times, then forward. Do this periodically, until you train your body back into a normal, relaxed posture. (If you reframe the message by telling yourself to lift up your collarbones, your shoulders will drop automatically.)

ENERGY DRAIN

The ear is loaded with acupressure points, which can relax and energize the entire body. Use lotion and massage your ears between your thumb and index finger, from bottom to top, and back down again.

IT'S A WASHOUT!

Mix a creamy, pearlescent eye shadow in pink or bronze in your palm with your foundation or moisturizer and apply to cheeks.

SWEATY PALMS

If you get sweaty palms when you're nervous or stressed, let four tea bags steep in 3 cups of hot water and cool. Dip a washcloth in the tea, and apply to palms for 15 minutes. The tannic acid in tea helps control the sweat.

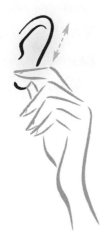

The ear is a sensitive organ on the outside, too.

stress-busting baths

And Skin Soothers, too!

When your stress muscles are flexing, there's nothing like sinking into a warm bath, where cozy comfort—and therapeutic treatments—will float your stress away. If you have time, luxuriate in a 15- to 20-minute soak (make sure to moisturize afterward or use bath oils in the bath to prevent dry skin), using one of the treatments opposite. If you don't have 20 minutes, even a 5-minute mini-soak can be relaxing. Here are a few tips on how to relax in the tub and fix stress-related skin problems at the same time.

Dull, Flaky Skin?
Mix a palmful of body wash with a small scoop of bath salts in your palm. Massage gently into your skin.

Oily Skin?
Cut two oranges in half, and squeeze into bath.

BATH TYPE	INGREDIENTS	WHY IT WORKS	TIPS FOR USING
Restorative	Mud	Mud is rich in minerals.	Mud warms the body and balances the skin's pH.
Moisturizing	Rice milk, soy milk, oat milk	Milk softens and soothes skin.	Especially good for sensitive skin.
Relaxing	Lavender	Lowers your cortisol.	Wait until the water stops running, then swirl oils through.
Rejuvenating	Rosemary, mint, citrus, ginger	Their scent revs up the circulation.	Before bath, massage a handful of bath salts into skin to exfoliate.
Stimulating	Sea salt	Salt stimulates the circulation.	Moisten sea salt or kosher salt, and rub it *gently* on your body, avoiding the face, neck, breasts, and any broken skin. Soak in a warm bath. Make sure to moisturize afterward.
Muscle Soothing	Epsom salts	Soothes sore muscles.	Sprinkle in a drop or two of eucalyptus oil to warm those muscles as well.
Anti-Itch	Colloidal oatmeal	The pasty, milky quality soothes skin and counters the itch.	Open a pack of Aveeno or place a handful of any oatmeal in a cotton sock, and hang it over the faucet so the water runs over it.

Dry Skin?

Run a warm—not hot—bath, and add 2 tablespoons of honey under the running tap.

Super-Dry Skin?

Add a cup of nonfat dry milk.

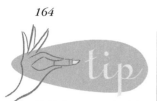

EXTREME ZIT

If you've got a big event like a wedding, graduation, or reunion coming up, and you wake up with a monster zit, here is a foolproof, extreme fast fix: Go to your dermatologist for a cortisone shot, which will eliminate the offender in under 12 hours.

LOCKLUSTER

Hair spray adds subtle shine. For super sheen, try this: Spray your hair with hair spray, then dip a pouffy powder brush into bronzing powder or gold or bronze eye shadow, depending on the color of your hair or your highlights. Shake the brush to get rid of the excess, and brush onto your hair, back from the hairline, concentrating on the roots.

SOOTHE TIRED EYES

Soak cotton pads in iced tea and apply to your eyes for ten minutes. Or try a portable depuffing eye mask. Pop one in the hotel minibar to help chill out from jet lag, or keep it in the fridge at home when you need to soothe tired eyes. These also take down surgery-related swelling.

PRODUCTS: Pearl Ice Cooling Mask by Inka ■ Talika Eye Therapy Patch.

PUFFY STUFF

If you wake up puffy, run an ice cube around your face on your way out the door. Cold has a contracting, toning effect, which is why it's also a good idea to keep your eye cream in the fridge.

ROSACEA ROADBURN

When rosacea makes your skin too sensitive for everyday makeup, try mineral makeup.

PRODUCT: Bare Escentuals Bare Minerals.

CODE RED

When your skin looks irritated and inflamed, and you see small red blood vessels and bumps that look like pimples, it may be rosacea. See your dermatologist, but in the meantime, drink green tea, which helps to calm inflammation. And look for skin creams with extracts of green or white tea, licorice (glycyrrhizinate), grapeseed, allantoin, resveratrol from red grapes, zinc, beta hydroxy acids, vitamin K and copper.

PRODUCTS: Replenix CF Cream ▪ Clinique CX Redness Relief Cream ▪ Eucerin Redness Relief ▪ Eau Thermale Avène Cream for Intolerant Skin.

COVER UP

To cover rosacea, look for "luminous makeup" (which diffuses light on the surface of the skin) or concealer and foundation with yellow undertones to neutralize the red. Use a damp sponge when applying makeup, and toss the sponge after each use.

PRODUCTS: Laura Mercier Secret Camouflage ▪ Lorac Illuminating Makeup ▪ Affirm Foundation.

ECZEMA

Eczema results in dryness, itching, flakiness, redness, and, occasionally, crusty blisters. Look for moisturizers with green tea, shea butter, borage oil, cortisone, jewelweed, or calendula.

PRODUCTS: Osmotics Tricerum ▪ Therapy Systems Emergency Treatment Cream ▪ Eau Thermale Avène Spring Water Soothing Serum ▪ Epoch Calming Touch Soothing Skin Cream.

FOR MORE HELP

For information on rosacea, check out the National Rosacea Society (www.rosacea.org) or the American Academy of Dermatology (www.aad.org).

secrets from the spaaaaah

The growth of the spa industry is a direct response to the overwhelming amount of stress in our lives. Massage therapists, aestheticians, and yoga and meditation teachers are all trained to help you relax, and a visit to a spa can provide a welcome antidote to stress. But if you don't have the time or money to go on a spa retreat, here are the favorite stress-relieving tips from directors of top spas around the country. *Do* try these at home.

Ginger Snap

Whip up a fresh ginger body scrub, suggests Shana Ominsky, of Claremont Resort and Spa, to recharge your batteries when they're running low. Grate a few stalks of fresh ginger and combine with an equal amount of coconut oil. Warm in the microwave for a minute, and when it cools, stir in a handful of raw sugar. Rub the mixture over your damp body from the neck down, then rinse off in the shower with lukewarm water. "Ginger stimulates the skin and brings blood to the surface," says Ominsky, "and the sugar acts as an exfoliant, leaving your body both invigorated and silky-smooth."

An Aromatherapy Moment

To ease the transition from a stressful day at work to a relaxing evening at home, Deborah Zie, of Cal-a-Vie spa, suggests that you light a few scented candles and dab some rosemary (or lavender or rose) essential oil on your pulse points—wrists, temples, behind the knees. "Turn off the phone, sit in your favorite chair, and breathe deeply to clear your mind of clutter," says Zie. "Try and let go of everything."

Mini Spa Retreat

"An hour before bedtime, take a relaxing herbal bath with essential oils of ylang-ylang and rose," says Barbara Close, of Naturopathica Holistic Health Spa. "Turn off the telephone and slip under the covers early with health and fitness magazines to inspire you for the next day," she continues. When you wake up, start your day with a facial sauna. "Heat a kettle of water. Fill the bathroom sink with the water and add four or five drops of clarifying essential oils such as juniper, petitgrain, or lavender. Place your head under a towel, lean over the sink, breathe in and relax."

Fast Foot Ritual

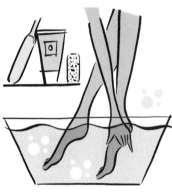

"Feet work so hard, and they're so neglected," says Laura Hittleman of Canyon Ranch spa. The antidote is a relaxing foot ritual in the evening before bed: Soak your feet in a basin of warm water, then smooth off any rough skin with a pumice stone or pedicure file. Massage a rich foot cream, such as MD Formulations Pedicreme, into the arches, between the toes, and on top of your feet. "Really slather it on," she says.

Good Intentions

When their stay at the Golden Door spa is over, guests are asked to "create a list of things they can do to relieve stress when they get back home," says Cindi Peterson, a behavioral therapist at the spa. Good things to have on your list are "time-outs" for a ten-minute meditation, nurturing yourself with a deliciously scented shower gel each morning, going for a facial, or practicing some deep belly breaths when the stress level is high. What would be on your list? Take a minute to make a list, and check things off as you do them.

more...secrets from the spaaa

Hawaiian Head Rush

This treatment offers a double benefit. "It is deeply nourishing and moisturizing to the hair and scalp and also helps to eliminate tension headaches and stress," says Emma Jayne Wright of the Kahala Mandarin Oriental spa. First, apply warm kukui nut oil (heat in microwave for about 15 seconds) to your scalp. (Use coconut oil if kukui nut oil is not available.) Separate your hair into sections and, using your fingertips, massage the oil into the scalp, working from the front of the hairline to the back. With spread fingers, apply firm circular pressure: Focus on moving the scalp, not the hair. Then comb through your hair with your fingers and wrap it in a towel. Run a hot bath (for steam) to help the oil absorb into the hair, and relax for 15 minutes. Shampoo and rinse.

A Virtual Vacation

"A quick, five-minute visualization can provide the little escape that you need to get through a hectic day," says Jennifer Cikaluk, of Kara Spa at the Park Hyatt Los Angeles. "On my desk I have a small photo of a sand dune in Mongolia that I once visited. It's a place of total balance and beauty. Whenever I'm feeling overwhelmed, I take a few minutes to stare at it and reground myself." To create your own visualization, Cikaluk recommends that you find an image that makes you feel peaceful, look at it for a while, then close your eyes, take some deep breaths, and mentally transport yourself to that place. Before you know it, you'll smell the sea air, feel caressed by the breeze, and your mind and body will relax.

office stress

Workplace-related stress costs the nation over $300 billion each year, according to the American Institute of Stress. That includes the cost of missed workdays and corporate funding for the burgeoning cottage industry that has sprung up to help employees deal with the fallout from downsizing, outsourcing, competition, long hours, no "downtime" due to instant global communication, and pressure to perform.

About 20 percent of employers nationwide have a stress-reduction program in place, according to *The New York Times*. It may not be surprising that the groovy Armani Exchange offers free yoga and meditation classes to employees, but when the straight-laced corporate management at AT&T does it, the message is clear: We must really be stressed out. If your company is not yet enlightened, here are a few ways to manage stress at the office on your own.

STRESS SPASM

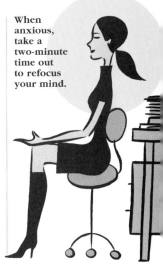

When anxious, take a two-minute time out to refocus your mind.

If you're heading into an important meeting and feel the choke grip of anxiety, duck into your office or an empty conference room. Sit with your feet hip-distance apart. Place your hands on your knees, palms up, close your eyes, and take a deep breath. Count to five as you inhale through your nose and again as you exhale through your mouth. (Make sure that your shoulders are down and back.) Repeat. On your next inhalation, hold your breath for five counts and exhale for five counts. Your body will relax, your mind will be focused, and you'll be ready to "knock 'em dead."

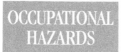

OCCUPATIONAL HAZARDS

Bad Air. Many office buildings are sealed environments, which means there's no fresh air circulating. What's worse, offices often contain toxins, such as the volatile compounds emanating from carpets, paint, copy machines, and computers.

Buy some plants for your office. Philodendrons, spider plants, cactus, English ivy, and peace lilies are actually capable of soaking up air pollution and toxins.

Bad Lighting. Fluorescent lights put strain on your eyes and can give you a headache. Bring in an incandescent lamp from home.

KAROSHI

The Japanese use the term *karoshi* to mean "death from overwork." But U.S. workers put in more hours on the job than even the Japanese, according to the International Labour Office. Take a tip from corporations in Japan, which enforce ten-minute exercise breaks at work. Close your door and do ten minutes of jumping jacks or stretches. Or get up and take a brisk walk or jog. Your endorphins will kick in, and you'll feel better almost immediately.

UPPER BACK TENSION

If your upper back is tense from hunching over your computer, stand up with your arms at your sides and slowly roll your shoulders back ten times, then forward ten times to loosen the tension in your muscles. Do it slowly and try to pinch your scapulae together as you roll back. Clasp your hands behind your lower back, and stretch your arms straight out behind you.

CYBER SORE

People who spend hours staring at the computer screen are more likely to develop eyestrain, sore back, even anxiety and insomnia. Give yourself a break and change your position every ten or 15 minutes. Look away from the screen toward some point in the distance to refocus your eyes. Take a brief walk once every 45 minutes to get your blood circulating and clear your head (get some fresh air, if possible).

DRY EYES

Working on a computer can make dry eye conditions worse because you blink less. Blinking remoistens the eyes and helps flush out dust and debris. Apply a warm compress to the eyes, especially around the tear ducts, several times a day. And try moisturizing eye drops.

PRODUCTS: Refresh ■ Theratears.

THE 4 P.M. FADES

Rinse or spritz your face with cool water, pinching your skin as you go. You'll see the color slowly return to your cheeks. Keep a small jar of gel—chilled aloe or a gel moisturizer—in the fridge at work. Pat gently on your face.

FALLING ASLEEP ON THE JOB

Close the door to your office (or use an empty conference room). Shake your arms, then your legs. Take a deep breath, and slowly bend over at the waist. Hang there for a minute or two, and then slowly, vertebra by vertebra, rise up to a standing position.

WANDERING MIND

Stand up, put your feet together, and rise up on your toes. Hold the position for about 60 seconds. Repeat five times. To maintain your balance in this exercise, you must concentrate your mind fully. That calms the mind so you can refocus on your work.

I sometimes see spots after staring at my computer screen. What should I do?

These are "floaters"—bits of protein in the vitreous humor of your eyes that become noticeable when you've been staring at something with a light background for too long. Check with your eye doctor in case it's something serious like a detached retina. Make sure to look away from your computer every 15 minutes to give your eyes a rest.

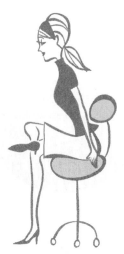

TIRED TOOTSIES

If you've been standing for a while and your feet are sore, sit at your desk, slip out of your shoes, and roll your feet back and forth over a tennis ball. It feels good, and creates an overall feeling of relaxation by stimulating acupressure points in the feet.

STIFF LEGS

Sit up straight, and cross your right ankle over your left thigh. Lean forward until you feel a stretch in your hip. Hold the position for a few seconds, then do it with the other leg. Get up and take a short walk.

CONTACT LENSES

If your eyes are sensitive, and they itch or tear up when you wear makeup with your lenses—especially in a dry office environment with fluorescent lights—here are a few makeup tips.

■ Put your lenses in before you apply eye makeup, and take them out before you remove your makeup.

■ Don't line the inner rims of your lids. Makeup can get trapped beneath your lenses and irritate your eyes.

■ Avoid cream eye shadow, which can melt and slip into your eyes. If it rubs against your lids, it can cause a sty.

■ Iridescent eye shadow, or other eye shadow with mica, may irritate your eyes. Read the label.

■ Avoid cotton puffs and Q-tips, except for the hard-pressed variety. Stray fibers can get into your eyes, and they're especially irritating to contact lens wearers.

■ Stick with pressed powders and pencils, because the warmth and oils from your skin can slide liquid liner and creamy eye shadows into your eyes, and loose powder can flake.

bottom drawer beauty

T o keep yourself looking fresh throughout the day—or to make that last-minute transformation from day to night when you're heading straight from the office out on a date—stash these items in your bottom desk drawer:

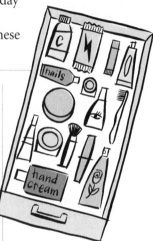

Create an oasis of comfort in your desk drawer.

■ **Concealer** to touch up the undereye area and any other spots—the area around the nose or blemishes—that need coverage

■ **Powder, blotting papers, a mattifier,** or **a shine stick** to tone down the 4 P.M. shine

■ **Blush** and **lip tint** to give you back some color, especially if it's been fading under fluorescent lights

■ **Toothbrush, toothpaste,** and **mini mouthwash**

■ A mini spray bottle of **rose water** or mineral water to hydrate your skin

■ **Eye drops**, especially if you get that bloodshot "Dawn of the Dead" look from staring at the computer screen

■ **Lip balm** for dry lips

■ **Hand cream** to apply throughout the day—make it a habit

■ **Cuticle softener** to massage into your cuticles (make a habit of doing this while you're on the phone)

■ A sample-size jar of **moisturizer** to pat on areas that have been dehydrated by dry air

■ **Packs of Emergen-C** when you need an energy kick or want to boost your immune system if colleagues around you are getting colds

■ **Low-fat protein-rich energy bars** and **mint gum** for those midafternoon munchies

PARCHED

Sitting near an old radiator all day can result in parched skin and hair. Put a pan of water on the radiator. Fill a mini spray bottle with water and keep it on your desk. (If your skin is oily, squeeze a few drops of lemon juice into it.) Spray your face, blot gently with a tissue, and repeat throughout the day. Your skin will look (and feel) refreshed.

SLEEPY FINGERS AND TOES

While sitting at your desk, wiggle your fingers and your toes, which will stimulate the circulation.

THROUGH A GLASS, DARKLY

You love the look of your lashes with mascara, but the tips sometimes touch the lenses of your glasses and leave little paw prints. After you apply mascara, touch the ends lightly with a tiny pat of powder.

BaD HaBITS

In addition to external stress, we also suffer lifestyle stress that results from bad habits—smoking; eating too many salty, sugary, or overprocessed foods; overdrinking, to name a few. Maybe you've partied too much in an attempt to escape your stress, and find yourself at work the next morning in a fog. Remember, just because you feel polluted doesn't mean you have to look that way.

CIGARETTE SMOKE

Tobacco smoke contains more than 4,000 chemicals, including carbon monoxide, formaldehyde, and benzene—and I don't need to tell you the severe health hazards. Smoke also stresses the skin; a heavy smoker is five times more likely to be wrinkled than a nonsmoker. Simply put, don't smoke! But if you do, laminaria digitata—a seaweed-based skincare ingredient—may help protect your skin from excessive damage, including that from secondhand smoke. Or, use an antioxidant cream to protect your skin from free radical damage.

BOOZER BLUES

Alcohol dehydrates the skin, makes wrinkles and puffiness more pronounced, and dilates the blood vessels, which can leave skin splotchy and stippled with small red veins. Drink water alongside your wine, which will not only slow you down, it will dilute the effects of the alcohol. Strengthen your capillary walls by getting your daily dose of vitamin C. Laser treatments administered by a dermatologist are the quickest way to repair broken capillaries.

HANGOVER HELPER

Mix a packet of Emergen-C, an energizing vitamin mix available at the health-food stores, into a tall glass of water and drink it down. For nausea, try a cup of chamomile or peppermint tea and avoid coffee, acidic juices, and fatty foods.

OVERSLEPT? FIVE-MINUTE WASH 'N GO

All of us need to catch up on our beauty sleep now and then—but not on a weeknight. If you *do* oversleep, it helps to have a plan:

1. Splash a few handfuls of cold water on your face. And pinch your face to make the color rise in your cheeks.

2. Dab some concealer (no time for foundation) just where you need it—under the eyes or on blemishes—and blend well.

3. Pull your hair back in a ponytail or twist.

4. Dab a bit of lipstick or gloss on your lips and cheeks and go!

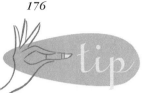

BLOODSHOT LIDS

After a late night, make a compress with cool raspberry tea, and apply it to closed eyes for five or ten minutes.

LASH LEFTOVERS

You're running late, and you don't have time to redo last night's leftover mascara. Wipe away any smudges under the eyes with a washcloth, and just touch the wand to the tips of the lashes for a hint of fullness.

PATCH FOR PUFFY EYES

Try a stick-on undereye patch infused with gels and plant extracts like chamomile, cucumber, mint, and aloe. Chill in the fridge overnight, and apply for approximately ten minutes in the morning.

PRODUCTS: Talika Eye Therapy Patch ▪ Chanel Precision Eye Patch Total ▪ Earth Therapeutics Hydrogel Under-Eye Recovery Patch.

PILLOW CREASES

If you've slept badly and wake up with creases on your cheeks, wash with warm water, then massage your cheeks with moisturizer for a few minutes.

NEED YOUR BEAUTY SLEEP?

According to the National Sleep Foundation, 74 percent of Americans have problems sleeping several times a week. Dab a drop of lavender essential oil on each temple before you go to bed. Or, mix lavender or neroli into a mini spray bottle half-filled with water, and spray your pillow (from a distance). When you lie down, the scent will tell your brain to relax, and before you know it, zzzz!

MEDICATIONS:

WHAT YOUR DOCTOR DOESN'T TELL YOU

Let's face it: We live in a pill-popping culture. At any given moment, nine out of ten Americans are consuming some form of over-the-counter or prescription drug—many of them having to do with our need to self-medicate our stress-related ills.

Most doctors don't bother to mention (or don't know about) the beauty fallout that can result from living in the land of meds. A number of medications can cause less-talked-about but still problematic side effects on skin, hair, energy, and sex drive. For example, did you know that antihistamines can parch your hair, antidepressants can make your skin look dull, and antibiotics can result in yeast infections and hyperpigmentation? Your doctor may not care about the effect on your looks from medications, but you should! Here is some side-effect information that I gleaned from talking to dermatologists, aestheticians, pharmacologists, and facialists. So guard against these potential problems when you take these drugs.

ANTIBIOTICS

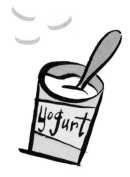

"Antibiotics can be very drying both inside and out, and yeast infections can result," says Kimberly Sayer, an aesthetician at the Affinia Wellness Spa in Manhattan. Sayer advises her clients to eat yogurt with acidophilus (a bacteria that neutralizes yeast) daily or take acidophilus capsules or powder while on antibiotics, and apply a moisturizing mask to hydrate dry skin.

TOUGH AS NAILS

If your nails seem weak and split since you've started your antidepressant prescription, massage neem oil into the nails and, especially, the nail bed.

PRODUCTS: Dr. Hauschka Neem Nail Oil Pen ▪ Sundari Neem Essential Oil.

Antibiotics make your skin sensitive to the sun, which can cause dark spots or hyperpigmentation. If you are on antibiotics, wear an SPF 15 sunscreen with zinc oxide or titanium dioxide whenever you head outdoors. If you see hyperpigmentation occurring, try a glycolic acid or calendula cream, which may slowly fade the spots. If they are stubborn, consult your dermatologist, and ask about a chemical peel or prescription fade cream.

PRODUCTS: Kimberly Sayer of London Tangerine and Calendula Healing Light Night Cream ▪ MD Formulations Vit-A-Plus Body Illuminating Creme.

ANTIDEPRESSANTS

"Antidepressants—i.e., serotonin inhibitors like Wellbutrin and Zoloft—can make the skin and hair look lackluster," says Dr. Jeanine Downie, author of *Beautiful Skin of Color*. Lightly exfoliate the skin two or three times a week to slough off the top layer, then follow it with a clay mask. Antidepressants may also cause really depressing side effects like hair loss, acne, and psoriasis, not to mention lowered libido. If you experience these, ask your doctor to switch you to another medication.

COLD MEDICINES

Over-the-counter cold medications, especially antihistamines, can dry out your skin and hair, just like they dry up congestion. Take flaxseed oil or sprinkle a teaspoon of flaxseeds on your yogurt or cereal daily. Moisturize your skin with a shea butter cream and massage or comb shea butter into dry hair before shampooing, cover with a warm towel for ten minutes, then shampoo.

ORAL CONTRACEPTIVES

Oral contraceptives have one famous side effect: They can clear up acne. In fact, Ortho Tri-Cyclen gained FDA approval to market their birth-control pill as an acne treatment. "Birth-control pills clear up your skin but it sometimes takes three months because the acne can flare up before it calms down," says Dr. Carol Livoti, coauthor of *Vaginas: An Owner's Manual.*

The pill can make some people appear puffy. If this happens, decrease your salt intake, drink lots of water, and sleep on two pillows. To reduce puffiness, lie down for five or ten minutes with a chilled gel mask or a bag of frozen blueberries on your face.

HORMONE REPLACEMENT THERAPY

Opinion is fiercely divided over whether hormone replacement therapy should be a recommended treatment for women with symptoms of menopause. But no one is arguing over that fact that it does make your skin look better. "Estrogen stimulates the connective tissue and thickens the skin," says Dr. Carol Livoti. "It will improve crepey fine lines and wrinkles, and it strengthens your bones."

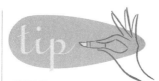

SUPER SOFTENER

Look for whipped shea butter, which is especially soft and penetrates really well, when your skin is really dry.

Q

*Why am
I losing
my hair?*

A

Stress and med-
ications like
barbiturates and
antidepressants,
may lead to hair
loss in women
(called androgenic
alopecia).
Treatments
include: topical
Rogaine (the 5
percent solution
for men is often
given to women
under a doctor's
care) the birth-
control pill, which
can help stimulate
hair growth;
antiandrogenic
drugs, which
block testosterone
receptors; and
certain vitamins,
like biotin.

STEROIDS

Steroids can lead to greasy hair, weight gain, and purple stretch marks and "they can cause what's known as a steroid acne," says Manhattan dermatologist Dr. Diane Berson, "which is most common on the chest and back." If the acne is not terribly severe, wash with a salicylic acid cleanser, and apply a clay mask to your chest and back three times a week. If you develop cystic acne, visit your dermatologist.

Oral steroids like prednisone and dexamethasone can cause the capillaries under the skin's surface to dilate, which can result in redness and flushing. Take soothing Aveeno oat baths, and look for skin creams with chamomile, lavender, vitamin K or licorice extract (glycyrrhizinate).

ANTISEIZURE MEDICATION

Antiseizure medication and schizophrenia medication can cause hair loss and acne. If the acne is severe—and it can be—ask your doctor whether you can switch to another medication.

CHEMOTHERAPY AND RADIATION

It may seem odd to be talking about cancer in a book on beauty. But the side effects of cancer treatments can have a devastating effect on appearance. Women battling the disease have enough to deal with already, without feeling unattractive, too. I know, from several family members who recently went through radiation and chemotherapy, that hair loss, skin problems, and scars from surgery can be demoralizing and debilitating. Plus, a beauty remedy might be one of the few small things you can do to help yourself or a friend feel better at a time when you or she has so little control over life's circumstances. So if you know someone going through chemotherapy, get informed. Below are some suggestions that will help ease appearance-related concerns and perhaps help a loved one get through an extremely difficult time—in style.

HAIR LOSS

Chemotherapy doesn't just stop cancer cells from dividing; it can stop the function of other cells like those in hair follicles, which may result in the loss of hair on your head as well as elsewhere on the body. Certain types of drugs—Cytoxan, Oncovin, and Adriamycin—cause the greatest hair loss, but the degree of hair loss depends on your dosage and varies from person to person.

Losing your hair can be traumatic—even though it does grow back—which is why some women pre-empt the process by cutting their hair really, really short or even shaving their heads before beginning chemotherapy treatments.

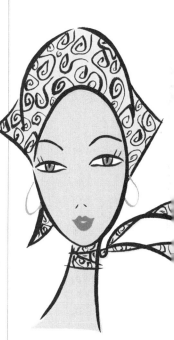

You can wrap an oversize scarf as a turban, or fasten it at the nape with a brooch.

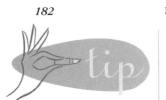

FAST FIX

Hair extensions and hair weaves will make your hair look thicker as it's growing back. And the right choice of hair color can make thin hair look a lot thicker. For example, if you're a fair-skinned blonde consider becoming a redhead for a while.

Some women prefer to invest in a wardrobe of beautiful head scarves; others decide to go *au naturel.* A thoughtful gift to get for a friend at this time might be a beautiful hat or scarf. Or perhaps you might offer to go with her to shop for a wig. Go before treatment starts so that it's easier to match her hair's natural color and texture. Here are some things to be aware of: Synthetic wigs are easier to wash, cooler and more comfortable to wear, and less expensive, while real-hair wigs look more natural. Some insurance companies cover the cost of a wig during cancer treatment, and your local chapter of the American Cancer Society should carry wigs at reduced rates, or even offer them for loan.

ROYAL FLUSH

Chemotherapy can cause the skin to flush as a result of the capillaries dilating under the skin's surface. Your flush may last for a few minutes or several hours. If your flush lasts longer, or is accompanied by fever, pain, or discomfort, call your doctor.

ITCHY SCRATCHY

Radiation, chemotherapy, and cancer itself may cause localized or widespread itching—known medically as pruritus—throughout the body. Take soothing oatmeal baths in cool water with Aveeno. Wash your body with a gentle, unscented glycerin soap. Moisturize your skin with a light lotion for sensitive skin, sweet almond oil, or calamine lotion. Sprinkle the areas with corn starch—

not talcum powder, it's too abrasive. Avoid clothing that's tight or clings. If itching really drives you crazy, your doctor may prescribe a prescription steroid cream or antihistamine.

HYPERPIGMENTATION

Your skin may hyperpigment—darken or turn orange—as a result of certain types of chemotherapy. The darkening may be localized—elbows, knees, palms, and soles—or it may look like you've hopped a plane to Aruba and gotten yourself a tan.

Take special care to protect your skin from the sun during this time. Wear a hat outdoors and limit your sun exposure. Use a sunscreen with SPF 15, and make sure it has titanium dioxide or zinc oxide listed as an active ingredient.

PALE NAILS

Certain types of chemo drugs—especially paclitaxel and docetaxel—can cause horizontal white lines, called Beau's lines, to form across your fingernails. They'll go away, but in the meantime, relax and get a manicure. (Bring your own tools because your immune system is compromised at this time.)

RADIATION FALLOUT

During treatment, your skin is more sensitive and will be easily irritated and prone to blister or crack. Treat it very gently—no scrubbing with washcloths or

CHEMO SKIN TIPS

During chemotherapy, your skin thins and becomes flakier, itchier, and more sensitive than usual. You'll sweat less than you usually do, which will leave your skin drier. And you may be more vulnerable to skin infections. Try to avoid directly exposing your skin to extremes of temperature. Avoid bathing or showering in water that is too hot or too cold. Moisturize your body while your skin is still damp to help seal in the moisture. If your skin acts up throughout your treatment, consult your doctor.

CANCER CARE

The Internet is an incredible resource for up-to-the-minute information on cancer treatments, symptom management, support groups, and side effects. Here are a few of the best sites.

American Cancer Society.
Your first line of reference.
www.cancer.org

Gilda's Club. This is an incredibly nurturing support facility for cancer patients and their families. It's named after Gilda Radner, the comedienne who died of ovarian cancer.
www.gildasclub.org

Look Good, Feel Better. This organization offers women with cancer tools to feel better about their appearance. They offer free lessons on beauty techniques and send you home with a goodie bag.
www.lookgoodfeelbetter.org.

The Wellness Community. An online support group and information resource on mainstream and alternative treatments.
www.thewellnesscommunity.org

loofahs, no aggressive skincare products, no heavily scented products, no petroleum jelly, no heavy detergents. The skin may darken in areas where you've had treatment. If you have to shave, use an electric razor to avoid cuts. Small cuts from shaving can easily become infected, which can lead to problems. If your skin does anything unusual throughout your treatment—if it blisters, cracks, feels wet, or starts to shed—check with your doctor.

PART IV:

on the go

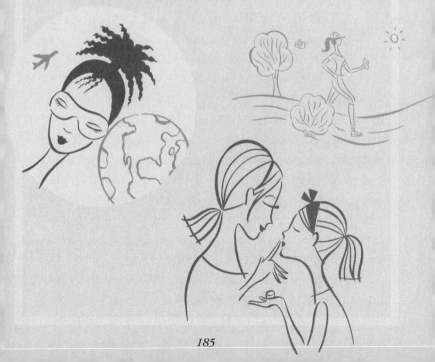

CHAPTER NINE

Travel

 OME OF US WERE BORN TO TRAVEL. FOR ME, IT'S LIKE falling in love—every time I get on a plane, it feels like the first time. Familiarity only makes it easier, never less thrilling.

Whether I'm traveling up the coast or across a few time zones, I rely on the locals for their expert advice on what to pack in my beauty bags. In England, the rainy, moist air keeps the skin naturally dewy, but it means that defrizzing products for the hair are definitely in order. In Phoenix, Santa Fe, and Denver, the mile-high city, the air is so parched that it saps every drop of moisture from the body. In other words, a thick, creamy moisturizer is mandatory. Since Australia has the highest rate of skin cancer in the world, you learn to take your sunscreen *very* seriously when you're down under.

Once you get the mechanics down—what to bring, how to pack, how to pinch-hit for what you leave behind—you'll find that you can focus on the romance of travel. This chapter will offer tips on how to smooth any bumps along the road.

En Route

If the prospect of packing your bags makes you feel emotionally overburdened, learn how to lighten the load. For all frequent business fliers, there's a cardinal rule of traveling light: Lay out everything you think you need on the bed, and then put half of it away before you pack. Be ruthless.

Choose fabrics that travel well so that your clothes don't look like they've been through the wringer when you arrive. Synthetic blends and light wools travel well. Silk, linen, and rayon don't.

NOTHING TO WEAR ONCE YOU GET THERE

Keep your color scheme consistent so you can mix and match and create more outfits with fewer items.

PRODUCT OVERLOAD

Collect "minis" whenever you can—mini toothpaste tubes, sample-size creams, even deodorant is downsized these days. (Scoop them up from your ritzy hotel for later or get them at most drugstores.) You can also buy small plastic travel jars and fill them with your own products. For a short trip, these will lighten your load considerably.

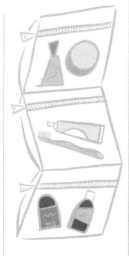

A clear, plastic make-up case saves time.

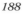

HOME AWAY FROM HOME

Pop a mini travel candle in your suitcase to scent your hotel room and make it feel cozier.

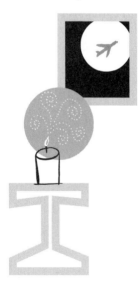

TAKING A SPILL

I learned my lesson when my perfume bottle broke at the beginning of an eight-hour flight. No more big breakables. Instead, I stock up on portable packets of makeup remover, nail-polish remover, face masks, and perfume samples. If you must carry bottles, seal in Ziploc bags!

PRODUCTS: Cutex Essential Care Advanced Nail Polish Remover Pads ■ Swabplus Eye Makeup Remover Swabs ■ Awake Vital Express Mask ■ Shu Uemura Moisture Face Mask (great, but pricey!).

PLANE TALK

The ideal humidity for healthy skin is 40 percent; airplane humidity hovers around 8 percent. Even a three-hour flight will suck every last drop of moisture out of your skin and hair. In addition, the stress of flying can trigger hormones that make the skin drier in some spots and oilier in others, resulting in flakiness, breakouts, and a dull, sallow complexion.

Knowing this, there are a few things I try to remember when on a plane:

Wear little or no makeup. Makeup dries out your skin even more on an airplane. Mascara can get messy, especially on an overnight flight. And, if you're prone to blackheads and clogged pores, you've probably discovered that your face tends to break out when you fly. To prevent travel breakouts, fly with clean, makeup-free skin and dab on moisturizer as needed en route. Just before you land, put on your makeup.

carry-on beauty

I've learned to travel with a little bag (inside my carry-on bag) filled with what I consider beauty essentials for air travel. They make the trip more pleasant, and you'll come out looking a lot better on the other end.

1. A bottle of water. You never know when you'll be able to catch the flight attendant's attention. Hydrate yourself from the inside out—you'll feel better, and your skin will look better, too.

2. A spritz bottle. Fill a mini spray bottle with water, add a couple of drops of lavender essential oil (or your personal favorite). Spray on your face and neck periodically throughout the flight to keep your skin hydrated. It feels good, it smells nice, and it really helps your skin.

PRODUCTS: Jurlique Aromamist Skin Refresher

Travel Blend ▪ Caudalie Beauty Elixir ▪ Eau Thermale Avene Thermale Spring Water ▪ Evian Spray.

3. A sample-size pot of face cream. Pat it around your face and under your eyes throughout the flight.

4. A sample-size pot of leave-in conditioner. Squeeze a dime-size dab of conditioner into your palm, rub your hands together, and lightly pat through your hair. Do the same with a dab of your moisturizer.

5. Eye drops that are not drying, like Refresh, to keep the eyes moist. Drugstores also carry whitening eye drops that shrink

the blood vessels and get the red out.

6. Hand wipes to avoid picking up germs from the airport or plane.

7. Packs of powdered vitamins to keep you healthy. Fashion stylists and models stock up on packs of Emergen-C (found at health-food stores) when they travel and need an extra boost of protection.

8. Lip balm to prevent lips from drying out.

9. Tic Tac mints or Supersmile In-Between Dry Mouthwash Crystals to freshen the breath immediately.

Limit alcohol and caffeine consumption. Both are diuretics and will dry out your skin. Also, the effect of alcohol is increased in the air. If you need a caffeine wake-up, or if you're a nervous flyer and need to fall asleep, go ahead and imbibe—just don't overdo it. If you drink too much alcohol or caffeine, you'll feel hung over or jumpy on the other end.

BeING THere

Some people like to create a home away from home when they travel, while others thrive on soaking up every shred of the exotic from their new environment. I fall squarely into the latter camp, but I do love to bring one or two cozy touches of home—a family photo, a mini-candle, a soft wrap for the plane—along with me.

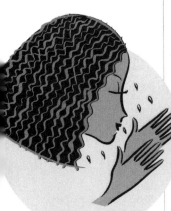

A splash of cool water is a great wake-up call.

THE MORNING AFTER

The morning after a night flight—or any flight—your skin may feel a bit peaked. Wash your face with a gentle scrub. Then alternately splash your face with cool, then warm, then cool water, four or five times. Apply a moisturizer that contains mint or rosemary. Dab a bit in front of your ears and on your wrists, and you'll feel instantly more alert.

SHUT EYE

After a long flight, it may seem that your eyes will never fully open. Stroke a light, neutral eye shadow over the top lid with a brush. Highlight your browbone with a paler shade, which will open up your eyes. Apply mascara in diagonal strokes toward the outer corners to extend your lashes outward.

- -

PRODUCT: Benefit Cosmetics Speed Brow Pencil.

THE RED EYE

Yellow neutralizes red. Apply a yellow-based concealer above and below the eyes close to the lashes. Eye shadow shades of gray, green, beige, and neutral brown will also tone down redness.

HOMESICK

To lift your mood (or freshen up your hotel room), spray perfume on one of your lightbulbs. The heat will diffuse the scent throughout your room.

UNRULY BROWS

To tame wild brows put hair spray or gel on your comb and run it through.

TOO MANY CONNECTING FLIGHTS

To perk up your skin after endless hours en route, chill a gel mask in your hotel minibar and apply it before you go to bed, followed by a rich moisturizer.

BREAKFAST IN BANGKOK?

If you've flown across the world for a business meeting with no time to nap, and

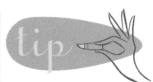

WRINKLE-FREE

Not your face, silly, your clothing. If you don't have a suit bag, lay your blouses and jackets flat, and place a dry cleaning bag on top. Then, roll your garment, like a sleeping bag, from the top to the bottom and pack it in your suitcase. The plastic will keep things wrinkle-free.

your skin looks as tired as you feel, run a disposable facial cloth around your face. It will moisturize and rejuvenate jet-lagged skin.

PRODUCTS: Neutrogena Hydrating Facial Cloth Mask ▪ Olay Skin Cleansers.

weaTHer RePorT

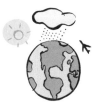

When you're traveling to different climate zones, you may not be prepared for what the weather has in store for you. Here are a few local experts' suggestions about what to expect and how to protect yourself from the elements.

HOT 'N HUMID

A little product know-how will keep your hair frizz-free.

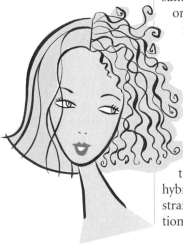

Anyone who has traveled to tropical climates like Rio or Bangkok, or spent a summer in New York City, Miami, Houston, or St. Louis, has seen how humidity can frizz the hair. To beat back frizz, "seal out the humidity with an antihumectant, which blocks the moisture from getting into your hair," says Mark Garrison of the eponymous Manhattan hair salon. He recommends this: For fine hair, use a spritz or two of hair spray, because it won't weigh down the hair. For medium, coarse, or curly hair, try a spray serum, an oil, or a serum/oil hybrid. For curly hair that's been blown straight, try a pomade, a leave-in conditioner, or a smoothing serum.

THE RAINY SEASON

In foggy, soggy climates like Seattle, San Francisco, or London, women are renowned for their fresh, flawless complexions. The moisture in the air keeps the skin naturally hydrated, but it can make a mess of your makeup. "In the foggy San Francisco climate," say Jean and Jane Ford, founders of Benefit Cosmetics, "it can be a challenge to keep your makeup looking fresh. Before you leave the house, be sure to dust a loose powder over your makeup. This will set your look and keep it from melting away in the morning mist."

POLLUTION

"Pollution breaks down the skin's immune mantle because of the free radical damage that it causes," says L.A. skincare expert Ole Henriksen, founder of Ole Henriksen Skin Care Center. "Irritating chemical residue makes up key components of pollution, and these particles have tiny molecules that readily absorb into human tissue and can cause rashes and irritation." Over time, it can also prematurely age the skin.

To reverse and neutralize damage, Henriksen suggests that you get your daily dose of antioxidants, especially vitamin C, bioflavinoids, beta carotene, and vitamin E, and drink at least one cup of green tea daily. Look for antioxidant creams to protect the skin daily, along with creams that contain noncomedogenic essential fatty acids like soy, grape, sesame, avocado, and rosa mosqueta.

SPA ALERT

If you're relaxing at a warm-weather spa or resort, factor in the sun when scheduling your spa treatments. For example, exfoliating treatments like body wraps, salt scrubs, body polishes, and peels expose a fresh layer of skin that is particularly vulnerable to UV light. Schedule those treatments for the end of the day. Exposure to chlorine, saltwater, sunscreen, and sand within a few hours of a treatment can also be irritating. Waxing right before sun exposure may make your skin more prone to a rash as can some essential oils used in aromatherapy treatments—especially citrus.

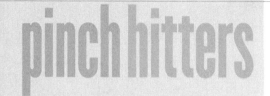

FUN PRODUCT SUBSTITUTES

We've all been there—it's 11 P.M., you've arrived at your destination and realize that even though your suitcases were stuffed well beyond the 70-pound limit, you've left behind something essential. Be clever, and pinch hit with something from your host's kitchen or substitute one product in your toiletries bag for another.

Left your Foundation at Home?

Mix a bit of **face powder** in with your moisturizer.

Forgot your Hair Conditioner?

Wash your hair, and substitute a squirt of **moisturizing lotion** for conditioner. Rinse well.

Eye Makeup Remover in your Other Bag?

Raid the kitchen for some **olive or vegetable oil** and dab it on a tissue to remove makeup. If your mascara is waterproof, try sesame oil on a tissue or cotton swab.

No Shampoo?

Use **shower gel**, which is shampoo for the body.

Need to Hand Wash Undergarments?

Shower gel or **shampoo** is gentle and effective for hand washing clothes.

No Body Lotion?

Use a dime-size dab of **hair conditioner** to moisturize hands, elbows, and feet—but *not* your face.

Close Shave?

Hair conditioner or **baby oil** are great shaving cream substitutes to use on your legs—they'll come out feeling silky and smooth.

No Hair Gel?

Run a bit of **shaving cream** through your hair. Just make sure that you use shaving cream, not shaving gel, which can get sticky.

No Blush?

Dab a bit of lipstick in your palm, and mix it with a bit of moisturizer. Apply it to your cheeks. Or, apply a pearlescent cream

eye shadow (pink or bronze, depending on your skin tone) to the apples of your cheeks.

Lose your Lipstick?

Mix a bit of **blush** in your palm with your lip balm and apply to your lips.

Need some Shine?

Pat a dab of **olive** or grapeseed **oil** through your hair. They add a natural sheen with no smell. (But not too much or you'll glisten like a plate of spaghetti carbonara.) Or, rinse your hair with a cup of brewed **Lipton tea**.

Got the Frizzies?

When your hair is frizzing, and you're without any defrizzing products, reach for the moisturizer. Or, take a dab of that **hand cream** you carry in your purse, pat it through your hair, pull your hair back, twist it, and pin it for a couple of minutes. When you take it down, you're frizz-free.

Forget your Face Cream?

Try **Cool Whip**. Sorbitol, a fatty alcohol that functions as a humectant in many moisturizers, is also an ingredient in Cool Whip. That's why, in a pinch, you can use Cool Whip to moisturize your skin and even condition your hair.

Stubborn Makeup?

If there's nothing else around, you can remove stubborn makeup the way theater people have done for ages—with **Crisco**!

Baby wipes will also do the job.

Your Dye's Showing?

If there's no hair-color stain remover around, remove hair-color stains from your hairline and forehead with **toner** or **milk**. Put a dab on a cotton pad and gently rub into the affected area.

Need a Diffuser?

Put a thin **sock** over the end of the dryer so your curls won't blow away. Next time before you pack, go to a beauty supply shop and buy a "sock"—a palm-size, spongy fabric attachment that's lightweight for traveling.

All Tied Up?

Use your **blow-dryer** to detangle your hair: Set it on cold and direct it at the tangles. Cold contracts the hair cuticle, which loosens the knot.

CHAPTER TEN

SPOrts anD THe GYm

B Y NOW, ANYONE WHO HASN'T BEEN LIVING IN A cave is aware of the benefits of exercise. In the short term, it makes you feel better almost immediately: Your endorphins kick in and elevate your mood. And you look better: Your heart rate increases, sends oxygen to your skin, and makes it glow. You sweat, which is the body's way of cleaning house and getting rid of waste. Your muscles strengthen and gain definition. Over time, exercise reduces your risk of disease, helps control your weight, focuses your mind, and keeps your heart healthy and strong.

In spite of all these great reasons to work up a sweat, most of us still don't get enough exercise. Unfortunately, the abstract benefits of exercise aren't enough to push us off the couch. That's why you have to find an exercise that you truly enjoy.

Exercise has to make you feel good *while* you're doing it. Maybe you like how buoyant and pain-free you feel in the water when you swim or the way the woods smell at different seasons when you hike. Maybe you enjoy the way a yoga pose makes your body feel alive with sensation. People who get hooked on these good feelings are the ones who stay with their exercise programs.

The most difficult thing about an exercise regime is getting started, and the second-most difficult thing is sticking with it. If you find yourself getting bored and making excuses, change the program: Vary your activity, bring a friend along, set a short-term goal, and work toward achieving it.

WORKING OUT

Being outdoors always makes a workout more enjoyable. A jog around the lake beats laps on an indoor track any day, just like a day out on the lake trumps the rowing machine. And there's no comparing an afternoon on the golf course with an indoor putting green.

HEAT FLUSH

Keep brewed green tea in a mini spray bottle in the fridge, and spritz it on your face to cool down overheated skin after an intensive workout. The tea is rich in anti-inflammatory polyphenols, and it will soothe your skin.

Just remember that it's crucial to wear a broad-spectrum SPF 15 sunscreen whenever you're outside. And one of the most important accessories for an active lifestyle is a bottle of water to keep you hydrated.

OPEN PORES

Before working up a sweat at the gym, which can clog pores and lead to breakouts, remove your foundation by washing your face or dabbing your skin with makeup remover or a moist towelette (see "The Gym Kit," page 204).

GLOW GOES

When you want to prolong your workout glow without makeup, spray your face with rose water when you get home to tone your skin (in summer, chill the rose water in the fridge). Then, apply a five-minute mask.

PRODUCTS: Aveda Intensive Hydrating Mask ■ Osea White Algae Mask ■ Kimberly Sayer of London Hydrating Antioxidant Facial Mask ■ Jurlique Deep Penetrating Cream Mask.

THE SWEATS

Moisture-wicking fabrics—especially in bras, shirts, and tank tops—keep you dryer and more comfortable during your workout and prevent you from getting a chill later. Wear clothes woven with nylon and supplex that wicks away sweat as you go. Online sources: www.danskin.com, www.usa.adidas.com, www.insport.com, www.nikewomen.com, www.nuala.puma.com.

MUSCLES IN A TWIST

When your muscles knot, apply arnica gel, cream, or oil.

PRODUCT: Naturopathica Arnica Muscle and Joint Bath and Body Oil

IN A BIND

If you eat less than 90 minutes before your workout, it will undermine the intensity, length, and calorie-burning potential of your exercise. A full stomach can also make you feel physically uncomfortable when you run, practice Pilates, or twist into certain yoga postures.

ENERGY FLAGS

Take a whiff of peppermint. Peppermint —in the form of gum, tea, oil, or scented lotion—will give you a boost.

WART-FREE YOGA

Just as you can pick up hepatitis when a manicurist uses unsanitary tools, you can get warts and athlete's foot from walking barefoot in the gym or yoga class. Invest in your own yoga mat (as well as your own manicure set).

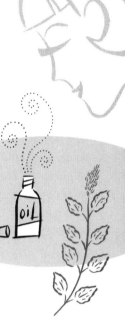

A peppermint Pick-Me-Up for low energy

WAXING RX

After waxing, don't use soap or astringent on the area for at least 24 hours, and avoid wearing tight pants or workout clothes that can irritate your skin.

SUPPORT YOUR TEAM

If you are a large-breasted woman and experience soreness during exercise, look for a sports bra with wide straps, which will give you extra support across your upper back and neck. When you try it on for fit and comfort, jump around in it to see if it provides the support you need.

EYE MAKEUP BREAKS DOWN IN A SWEAT

If you want your eye makeup to hold up through your workout, look for long-wearing water-based eye shadow (which can double as eyeliner). The color is smudge-proof for six to eight hours. Other formulations may be oily and can run as you sweat.

PRODUCTS: Maybelline Liquid Eyes Eye Shadow ■ Sue Devitt Studio Starlights Clear Water Eye Shadow.

FUNKY FEET

If possible, don't wear the same sneakers every day. It's a good idea to alternate your sneakers, giving them a chance to dry out so they won't harbor fungus.

ODORIFIC

Scent rises, especially in warm weather. Restrict your fragrance application to points south of your neck, especially when you're exercising indoors. Otherwise, you may overwhelm yourself—and your workout buddies—with too much of a good thing. Be considerate of others and don't wear scent in a closed environment like an exercise or yoga class.

ITCHY THIGHS

Ever find that when you exercise outdoors in winter, your thighs start to burn and itch? Sweat, friction, and the cold can combine to increase your sensitivity to synthetic fabrics. Try natural fibers like silk or wool.

Use fragrance-free and dye-free laundry detergent, and skip the fabric softener, which can leave irritating residue on your skin. The salt from your sweat may also be irritating dry skin. Shower immediately after your workout, pat your skin dry, and apply medicated powder.

SWEAT DRIPS

Sweat trickling down your face during a workout is not only embarrassing, it can be an annoying distraction. Wear a baseball cap or sweat band while you're working out. If you want something with more style, look for bandannas woven with moisture-wicking fibers.

THERE'S THE RUB

When you first take up cycling or spinning, you're bound to feel muscles—along with aches and pains—that you've never felt before. To ease the rub on your backside and the tender flesh between your thighs, get a gel seat and wear padded biking shorts.

SLUGGISH MUSCLES

To energize and warm your sore muscles, use a ginger body lotion, or grate a small piece of fresh ginger and mix it with a palmful of unscented body lotion. Massage into skin.

PRODUCTS: Origins Ginger Souffle ■ Pharmacopia Ginger Body Lotion ■ The Thymes Ginger Milk Body Lotion.

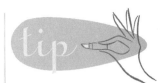

SHOWER SHORTCUT

If you don't have time to shower after a workout, wipe under your arms with baby wipes or towelettes.

Ginger snaps your energy.

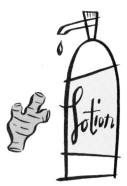

SWIMMER'S HAIR

If you're a swimmer and you're blond—especially if you color your hair—you know what you're up against when it comes to chlorine and your hair. The pool can turn your buttery blond to fright-night green, but here's how to prevent—or correct—the problem.

To prevent green hair, rinse your hair with club soda or seltzer as soon as you get out of the pool. Or, wash your hair with shampoo and rinse with V8 juice. It keeps the green out!

To get rid of green hair, massage ketchup, tomato juice, or tomato paste through wet hair. Leave it on for a couple of minutes, then rinse, shampoo, and condition as usual. Or, dissolve three aspirin in a cup of water, massage through wet hair, leave on for five minutes and rinse.

PRODUCTS: Green Out Shampoo ■ Suave Clarifying Shampoo ■ L'Oreal Kids Swim Shampoo,

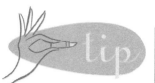

SOFT SMOOCH

To keep lips healthy, soft, and supple, pick up a portable tin of shea butter— a thick all-around moisturizer—and massage it into your lips before you apply gloss.

LIP TIP

Statistically, men are much more vulnerable to lip cancer than women. That's because titanium dioxide, the ingredient that gives lipstick its opacity, is also a broad-spectrum sunscreen. When you exercise outdoors, leave your lipstick on, or use an SPF 15 lip balm.

RABBIT-RED EYES

Wear goggles to protect your eyes from chlorine, but if your eyelids get red after swimming, it's easy to cover up. Try a cream concealer in a banana-based shade to tone down redness around the eyes.

PRODUCTS: Benefit Lemon-Aid ■ T. LeClerc Liquid Concealer (Banane)

SWIMMER'S EAR

It's important to keep your ear canal dry to prevent swimmer's ear. While drying your hair after swimming, give your ears a very quick blast from the blow-dryer, which will dry up any water, pronto! When the water is trapped in the canal, it exacerbates the growth of bacteria that live there and causes infection. (See your doctor if you develop pain or fever.)

GARDENER'S HANDS

If you love to garden but hate the inevitable dirt-clogged fingernails, run your nails along a cake of soap before you hit the vegetable garden. Your nails will clog up with soap, not dirt, and they will be easier to clean when you're done. Or, put on two layers of gloves: rubber gloves followed by gardening gloves.

DEEP STEAM

After your workout and shower, give your hair an intensive treatment while you relax in the steam room. Apply a deep conditioner to damp hair, cover it with a towel or shower cap if you like, sit in the steam for ten to 15 minutes, then rinse it out in the shower.

THIN RED LINES

Always apply a thin coat of moisturizer before you enter the sauna. It protects the skin from broken capillaries.

My lips get really chapped on the ski slopes, especially when I wear lip gloss. Why?

Wind and winter chill sap moisture from your lips. Even though lip gloss may make lips look moist and glossy, certain ingredients can actually dry them out. A thick, waxy lip balm—like ChapStick, Eau Thermale Avène Lip Balm with Cold Cream, or Kiehl's Lip Protector—will soothe lips and protect them from drying out in extremely cold weather.

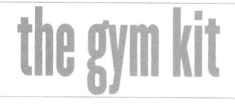

the gym kit

Start with a small case (with a handle, if possible), and fill it with travel-size toiletries. You can buy prepackaged minis—including individually packaged products for one-time or weekly use—at the drugstore, but it's less expensive, over the long run, to fill and refill your own little plastic containers with your favorite products.

Here's what you'll need:

Towelettes. Use these to remove makeup before your workout. Look for alcohol-free, botanical-infused towelettes without the antibacterial ingredient triclosan, which can irritate and overdry the skin. Makeup-remover and deodorant towelettes are also available.

PRODUCTS: Awake Cleansing Sheets ■ Comodynes Deodorant Towelettes ■ Herban Essentials Towelettes.

Deodorant. Buy it in the new mini-size.

Shampoo, conditioner, and shower gel. Pack these in easy-to-use mini squirt-top containers. And if you run out of shower gel, you can always wash your body with your shampoo.

Moisturizer. You'll need both face moisturizer and body lotion—all of that sweating can leave your skin dry.

Comb, brush, pony-tail elastic, or hair-styling products. Have these handy for giving damp hair a quick 'do.'

Sun protection. Before you head back outdoors, apply a moisturizer or sunscreen with SPF 15.

Flip-Flops. Don't go barefoot in the gym, and especially not in the shower, where you can pick up a case of athlete's foot. Keep a pair of flip-flops stashed in your gym bag.

Tissues. Just in case.

Toothbrush and toothpaste or mouthwash. When your mouth gets dry after a workout, this helps.

WORKOUT CRAMPS

If you're prone to leg cramps when you exercise, eat something salty like crackers and drink a small glass of water before you work out, then again when you're finished. You may also have a potassium deficiency. Eat a banana a day.

These may help prevent leg cramps.

POST-WORKOUT GRIME

Exercise can dehydrate the skin, and a soap-and-water combo can dry it out even more. If your skin is dry, don't wash your face with soap or cleanser after a workout. Instead, apply an alcohol-free toner—or use an alcohol-free towelette—to get rid of dirt and sweat.

WORKOUT BREAKOUT (BACNE)

When you wear tight workout clothes, sweat and friction—combined with your skin's natural oils—can lead to breakouts on your body, especially on your back. And if you're a hiker, it's not uncommon to get "bacne" from sweat trapped under your backpack. Here's how to avoid it:

▪ Take a shower right after your workout, and wash your back with a salicylic-acid body wash. Exfoliate with a scrub. Then, apply a salicylic-acid spot treatment.

▪ Apply a blemish-busting mask to your back (and chest, if necessary) two or three times a week.

▪ Wear natural-fiber clothing or sweat-wicking fabrics that will absorb sweat and keep it away from your body.

▪ Don't put on tight or fitted clothing until your back is clean and completely dry.

PRODUCTS: MD Formulations Alpha Beta Daily Body Peel (pads) ▪ Origins Spot Remover ▪ Neutrogena Body Clear Body Wash ▪ Benefit Cosmetics Bionic Blast ▪ Aveeno Clear Complexion Correcting Treatment.

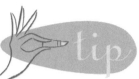

SLIM FAST

To make your bare legs look a bit slimmer, slick a bit of Johnson's Baby Oil Gel, Rosebud Salve, body oil, or even hair serum along your shins.

DRY SKIN, NO LOTION

Let's say you're at the gym without any body lotion. Hop in the shower and wash with conditioner, not soap. Rinse off, and see how silky you feel.

TEMPORARY LEG SLIMMER

Soak your legs in warm water and Epsom salts for a couple of minutes. Pat them dry, then apply a seaweed mask (seaweed is a diuretic, which means that it pulls water out), and wrap legs with Saran Wrap and a towel that's just warm from the dryer. Rest and relax for 15 minutes with your legs elevated, unwrap your legs, and rinse off the mask.

POLAR PODS

If the circulation in your feet tends toward sluggish after a freezing afternoon on the ski slopes or in the skating rink, warm your polar pods with a dab of menthol-based gel or balm or a peppermint moisturizer.

PRODUCTS: Blue Yoga Gel ■ Tiger Balm ■ Naturopathica Peppermint Tea Tree Foot Balm.

CHAFED BELLY

If your elastic waistband caused chafing on your belly or back, apply a cream with licorice extracts (glycyrrhizinates), which soothes minor irritation.

PRODUCTS: Eucerin Redness Relief Daily Perfecting Lotion ■ Soothing Care Chafing Relief Powder Gel.

ATHLETE'S FOOT

■ Apply a few drops of tea tree oil (available at the health-food store), a strong antibacterial and antifungal agent, directly to the area, or try a tea tree spray at least three times each day. (Tea tree oil has a strong odor, and if you prefer not to carry that with you, soak your feet in warm water spiked with tea tree oil at home in the morning and evening.)

■ Neem oil has a slightly less offensive odor, and also works quite well. Add a few drops of neem oil to a warm footbath. Soak for ten minutes or so.

■ An apple cider vinegar soak will also kill the fungus, but it may sting a bit.

■ Dry your feet, and apply medicated foot powder to your feet, especially between your toes—or massage with cornstarch before you put your socks on. Repeat several times a day for a couple of days until the condition clears up.

ALL WOUND UP

Try to work out at least two hours before bedtime. If you feel too hyped up and achy to sleep after your workout, run a warm bath and toss in a cup or two of Epsom salts, a quarter cup of soothing baking soda, and a relaxing lavender bath oil. Breathe in deeply, relax, and you'll sleep like a baby.

CRACKED CLAWS

After a day on the slopes, your chapped hands may need an intensive moisturizing treatment. Apply a thick layer of Bag Balm (or another rich hand cream) to your hands before you go to bed, and cover them with a pair of cotton gloves (they're cheap at art-supply stores).

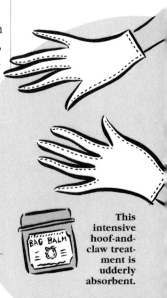

This intensive hoof-and-claw treatment is udderly absorbent.

PRODUCTS: Boscia Daily Hand Revival Therapy ■ Weleda Hautcreme ■ Jurlique Lavender (or Rose) Hand Cream.

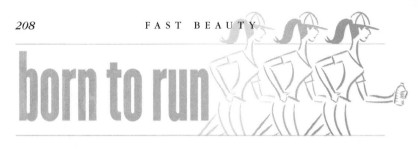

born to run

Here's a tip sheet of quick cures for common runner-related maladies.

Sayonara, Soreness

Do what the Japanese do: Soak your feet in hot water, then rub vigorously with a towel to stimulate circulation. Massage each toe three times in a clockwise, then counterclockwise direction. Then gently pull on each toe, place your foot in your lap, and massage the sole with your fists.

Achy Feet

Find a flat stone and heat it in the microwave for a minute until it feels warm but not hot. Massage the bottoms of your feet and between your toes with the stone until the achiness goes away—or the stone turns cold.

Side Stitch

Runners are prone to side cramps, triggered when the diaphragm spasms from all that heavy breathing. Slow your pace, take a couple of deep breaths, and gently massage the area. To prevent cramps, remember what Mom used to say: Don't eat an hour before you exercise. Also, sip, don't gulp, your water as you run, and breathe deeply from your diaphragm.

Achy Arches

If your arches ache, your plantar fascia (connective tissue from heel to toe) may be inflamed. Roll the arches of your bare feet back and forth over a can of frozen orange juice. The combo of cold and massage will soothe the inflammation.

Jogger's Nipple

Sore nipples are a common problem for both male and female long-distance runners. Jogger's nipple—soreness, dryness, inflammation, even bleeding —is caused by the friction of the nipple against clothes while you're running. Avoid close-fitting clothes in synthetic fabrics. Wear a silk or cotton bra. Apply shea butter, Vaseline, Band-Aids, zinc oxide cream, or nipple guards (intended for nursing women) before you head out for a run.

Jogger's Toe

This bruise beneath the nail (also called "tennis toe") results from the impact of your toes banging up against the toe box of your sneaker. Keep your nails trimmed, and get a pair of running shoes with a bigger toe box.

BLACK AND BLUES

Apply a vitamin K cream (phytonadione), available at the drugstore, to reduce bruising. (Cosmetic surgeons recommend topical vitamin K after surgery.)

PRODUCTS: Vita-K Solution for Scars & Bruises ■ Jason Vitamin K Cream ■ K Derm.

TO COVER A BRUISE, SCRATCH, OR SCAR

Use a stick concealer. Warm a dab in your palm (your body heat softens it and enables it to work into the skin better). With a small brush, apply it to the area. Pat it down with your fourth finger. Add another layer, if needed, and top with a light dusting of translucent powder.

TO FADE SCARS

Use a vitamin K cream twice a day and be patient—it can take from two to eight weeks. Or apply lavender essential oil directly to the scar. (Recent injuries heal faster than older ones.)

SUNSCREEN ON THE GREEN

If sunscreen makes your hands too slippery to control your golf clubs, use sunscreen pads instead of lotion or spray. They're neater to use, not at all greasy, and portable enough to reapply.

PRODUCTS: MD Formulations Sunscreen Pads with Vitamin C ■ Dermalogica SPF 15 Pads ■ Completely Bare Solar Shield SPF 30 Pads (oil-free).

What can I do to soothe sore muscles?

Soak in a warm (not hot) bath spiked with Dead Sea salts or Epsom salts to relax and soothe sore muscles after a workout. Epsom salts contain magnesium, which helps your body dispose of lactic acid deposits that cause the aches. And Dead Sea salts replace trace elements and electrolytes you've sweated out.

PRODUCTS: Burt's Bees Bath Crystals ■ Ahava Dead Sea Bath Salts.

CRACKING UP

Feet bear the brunt of almost 9,000 steps every day, which can be especially tough on your heels if you're carrying extra weight around or you're a runner. To soften cracked heels: Apply a moisturizing face mask. Cover with thin cotton socks for one to two hours. Repeat for several days as needed.

TIRED DOGS

Soak tired tootsies in a basin of lukewarm water spiked with mineral salts (available at a bath and body shop), Epsom salts, or, in a pinch, table salt. Shake in a few drops of eucalyptus or clove oil (if you don't have oil, crush a few cloves with a mortar and pestle and toss in your foot bath). The salts help your body dispose of lactic acid deposits; the oils stimulate blood flow and nerve endings.

INGROWN TOENAIL

Clip your nails straight across. Soak your foot in warm water to soften the nail. Gently lift the nail until you can slip a piece of cotton underneath, to keep it away from the skin. Do this for a couple of days, if necessary. If your ingrown nail becomes infected, see your doctor or a podiatrist.

BLISTERS

If you decide to run the Boston Marathon in a brand-new pair of sneakers, chances are you'll get a blister. Wash it with soap and water, and apply an antibiotic ointment to

To prevent ingrown toenails, clip nails straight across.

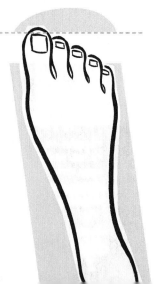

prevent infection. Leave it open to the air when you're home—it will heal more quickly.

CORNS

Apply a strip of lemon peel (with the inside against the corn), pineapple, or wet black tea bag and fasten with a Band-Aid. Leave on overnight and continue for a few nights until the corn goes away.

PRODUCT: J. Pickles Corns, Callouses & Hard Skin Ointment.

A FUNGUS AMONG US

Locker rooms, swimming pool perimeters, the inside of synthetic shoes, even a tight bandage on your toe can all harbor bacteria that cause nail fungus. If you share pedicure tools, you can share a fungus, too. Before you go to bed, apply Vicks Vaporub to your toenails. Cover with cotton socks and leave on overnight. (This remedy may take up to a week.) Or soak the nail in white vinegar once a day for several days. Supplement these treatments with a medicated foot powder, and wear it throughout the day.

YOU CALLOUS SOLE

Don't cut calluses, because they can get infected. Apply a foot cream with gly-colic acid, which will help slough off dead, callused skin.

PRODUCT: Luscious Foot Cream ■ MD Formulations Pedicreme.

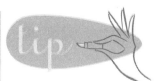

DANCING FEET

Look for foot moisturizers and foot soaks with mint, rosemary, eucalyptus, and citrus, which help rejuvenate tired feet.

sweet feet

E xfoliating the feet—and the hands— only takes a minute, and it really softens the skin. The soles of your feet are 20 times thicker than most other areas of the body, which is why you can use abrasive ingredients like salt, sugar, and cornmeal to slough off and soften them. Here are a few of my favorite ingredients to sweeten the feet.

Grapefruit. Fresh grapefruit is a tart, luscious exfoliant. Sit on the edge of the tub. Soak your feet in ankle-high cool water and rub sliced grapefruit over them. Massage sugar into your feet and dip them back into the cool water. After exfoliating, rinse the feet. Pat dry. Massage with a rich peppermint or citrus body or foot cream.

Lime. Try the same treatment, substituting sliced lime for grapefruit, and a handful of coarsely ground cornmeal for sugar.

Lemon or Blood Orange. Try the same treatment, with lemon or blood orange and salt. Add 3 tablespoons of olive oil to the soak.

Avocado. Avocado oil is extremely moisturizing and rich in vitamin E. After one of the above treatments, massage a small dab of avocado oil into your feet.

STEP LIVELY 7-MINUTE PEDICURE

I f you suffer from foot pain, take a few minutes to kick back and pamper your pods with a relaxing pedicure.

1) Exfoliate rough, dry skin with a pumice stone.

- - - - - - - - - - - - - - - -

2) Wet the feet and scrub with bath salts.

- - - - - - - - - - - - - - - -

3) Soak in warm water spiked with energizing peppermint or rosemary bath oil.

- - - - - - - - - - - - - - - -

4) Towel dry. Push back cuticles with an orangewood stick.

- - - - - - - - - - - - - - - -

5) Separate toes with tissue, put your feet up, and apply polish.

CHAPTER ELEVEN

your Family

ENTURIES AGO, LIFE LUMBERED ALONG AT A MUCH more leisurely pace than it does today. Indeed, extended families lived together under one roof, and folk wisdom was passed down from one generation to the next. Finding relief for a variety of ailments, and maintaining balance between body and spirit—what we call "wellness" today—were considered an intergenerational family affair. If your mother or great auntie didn't know what to do for a wart, a mosquito bite, or a dark moment of the soul, chances are your grandma did.

But these days, the nuclear or fractured family is more likely the norm. Separated by distance, divorce, or the pressures of daily life, each of us is more isolated and self-reliant. But that independence comes at a price—we don't always have the surefire answers that our grandmothers had at their fingertips. Of course, we do have the benefits of modern science and technology, but you'd be surprised at how many of those high-tech cures hail back to Grandma's folk wisdom. This chapter draws on a little bit of both to give you quick answers to some of the common ailments your family is likely to experience. (Because teens and tweens are going through such major physical transitions, they deserve their own chapter, see page 62.)

BABIES

Nature looks out for a newborn: When babies are born, their bodies are coated with a thick, waxy, yellow-white substance called vernix, which helps retain moisture in their skin and prevents it from drying out until their oil glands and pores start to function. Aside from the common conditions—cradle cap, diaper rash—most of the time, a healthy baby's skin and hair (little that there is!) is perfect. Here are the answers to simple questions about baby "beauty" care; anything more serious should be brought to the attention of your pediatrician.

DRYNESS AND CRACKING

Massage a bit of olive oil into your baby's hands, feet, wrists, and ankles to keep the skin from cracking until her own oil production system starts to function.

RASH DECISIONS

The most common causes of diaper rash are the skin's proximity to wet or soiled diapers, chemicals in the laundry detergent or disposable diapers, or a reaction to food or formula. To speed up healing, clean your baby's bottom and expose it to sunlight for up to ten minutes—even through a window. Then, apply a thick, occlusive ointment designed to heal diaper rash.

BABY BUMPS

Newborns sometimes develop tiny white bumps, called milia, on their noses and elsewhere on their bodies. Milia indicate that the baby's oil glands and pores are starting to function. Leave them alone, and they will go away, eventually, on their own.

CRADLE CAP

Cradle cap is a scaly crust that forms on some babies' heads, especially around the soft spot, from oil secretion. Shampoo once or twice a week with a diluted baby shampoo, and gently nudge the scaly skin off your baby's scalp with your finger as you wash. Or, heat some sweet almond or olive oil until it's lukewarm, *not* hot, and apply very gently to the affected areas. Don't rub.

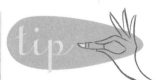

MOM'S MAKEUP

Mix a capful of your baby's no-tears baby shampoo into a cup of warm water and use it to tissue off your eye makeup.

Leave the oil on for about 30 minutes, shampoo the baby's head, gently massage the scalp, and rinse.

CRYING JAGS

Rub your child's tummy with rose water or a dab of vanilla extract. It will calm him down.

KIDS

Whether your child is suffering from a bruise, an interminable case of hiccups, or a bee sting, everyone in your household will benefit if you know what to do. Children can bounce back from almost any situation, and it helps if parents are resilient, too.

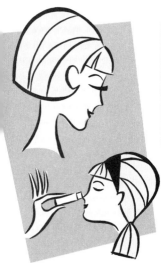

Learn good habits, like sunscreen, early on.

STICK-TO-IT SUN PROTECTION

For sun protection that stays where it should—on the ears, around the eyes—use a sun stick.

PRODUCTS: California Baby Sunblock Stick ▪ Dr. Hauschka Skin Care Sun Block Stick SPF 30 ▪ Clarins Sun Control Stick ▪ Mustela Sun Protection Stick.

WHAT WART?

Take a small piece of banana peel and place it against the wart with the inside of the peel facing the wart. Cover it with a Band-Aid. Leave it on around the clock and replace the Band-Aid daily, for a couple of days, until the wart is gone.

HICCUPS

Add a teaspoon of vinegar to a glass of water, and drink it slowly. Press down on your child's wrist where the pulse is, and hold to the count of 90. Or, have your child drink out of the opposite side of a half-full glass of water. (Kids have fun doing this, but it's best if they do it over the sink.)

TERRIBLE TANGLES

Wet the hair and work peanut butter through the tangles. Gently comb out the hair, starting at the ends and working up, to the roots. Shampoo and condition.

LICE SQUAD

Coat the hair well with mayonnaise or olive oil, and leave it in for half an hour. Shampoo with a tea tree oil shampoo, condition, and rinse well.

GUMMY HAIR

Wet the hair and apply a half cup of vinegar diluted in a cup of warm water to the area entangled in gum. Leave it on for a few minutes. The vinegar is acidic, which will cause the gum to break down. Comb through the hair, starting at the ends and working up to the roots, then shampoo.

HEY, BRUISER

To take the black and blue out of a bruise, wipe it down gently with rubbing alcohol.

What can I do about my son's prickly heat rash?

When sweat glands get clogged, it creates an itchy inflammation that looks like a cluster of tiny blisters. Apply cold compresses soaked in 1 cup of chamomile tea or water mixed with 2 teaspoons of witch hazel. Give your child a cool oatmeal or Aveeno bath. Calendula ointment or Benadryl will stop the itch. In warm weather, avoid dressing your child in synthetic fabrics.

PRODUCTS:
California Baby Calendula Cream
■ Aveeno Anti-Itch Gel Spray.

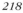

MUD CURE

Native Americans apply mud to bug bites to soothe the itch. If you're outdoors, scoop up some mud and dab it on the bite. If you're indoors, apply a dab of a clay mask (mother's mud) to the spot.

BUMPS AND BRUISES

Arnica gels or ointments (available at health-food stores) will ease the tenderness and take down the swelling caused by bumps and bruises.

BUZZ OFF

Bee stings are not only scary for kids, they hurt! Remove the stinger if you can. Then apply any of these remedies to soothe the sting: a thin layer of meat tenderizer, apple cider vinegar, mud, or a dab of honey (though that may seem counterintuitive).

Warning: Act fast and seek immediate medical attention if your child shows any of these signs of an allergic reaction to bee stings: difficulty breathing, generalized swelling, signs of shock, or any other symptoms that seem unusual.

HORNET STINGS

Remove the stinger if you can, cut an onion in half, and hold the onion against the sting for up to five minutes. Or, you can hold a slice of dill pickle against the sting. Really!

TOO MANY CHEMICALS

If you want to avoid chemical-based insect repellents, look for those made with essential oils like citronella, eucalyptus, lavender, and lemongrass, which will repel insects without potentially harmful ingredients.

PRODUCTS: Muti Oils Bug Away ■ Badger Anti-Bug Balm.

MOSQUITO BITES

Calamine lotion is, of course, the classic way to soothe an itch. Or, apply a bit of witch hazel to the bite. My grandfather used to mix a bit of sugar with water and put it on my mosquito bites. You can also place a chilled, brewed tea bag on the bite or a dab of toothpaste.

Simple household products are great multi-taskers, especially in a pinch.

A LONG DAY'S JOURNEY

A car ride with kids who are prone to car sickness may be the trip from hell. Ginger is an amazing antidote to nausea and car sickness. Keep ginger candies, lozenges, or tea handy in the car. Peppermint lozenges will also calm an unsettled, nauseous stomach.

CHICKEN LITTLE, BIG POX

Scratching chicken pox can lead to scarring. To prevent scratching and keep your child more comfortable, give her oatmeal baths. A soak in a cool Aveeno bath will soothe her skin. Or, fill a cotton sock or muslin sack with oatmeal, fasten the top with a rubber band, drop it in the tub as it fills with water, and give it a gentle squeeze now and then. Or, squeeze it against your child's skin to release the milk directly onto the affected areas.

PAPER CUT

If that school project led to a paper cut, clean it with soap and water. Apply Elmer's

a mom moment

Beauty Bonding

From an early age, little girls play with makeup. Who knows what makes turquoise eye shadow and orange nail polish so appealing to a five-year-old? Maybe they're drawn to color cosmetics for the same reason they're attracted to colored markers. It gives them an artistic outlet, and it's a way for them to express their creativity. Take

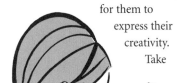

advantage of their interest, and use it as an opportunity to teach your daughters—or nieces, or friends' daughters—a healthy approach to skincare and beauty at a young age. This is the perfect opportunity for what I like to call a little "beauty bonding." When my daughter was in elementary school, we'd sit around the table (or in the bathroom) and make concoctions like body glitter and lip gloss.

Mixing up beauty products can be a great activity for kids. Why not invite a group of your daughter's friends over, sit around the kitchen table, and make some simple products?

Beauty bonding is fun, it makes great gifts, and it's a way to connect with your kids. It's also an inexpensive alternative to trolling the bins at Origins and The Body Shop— a favorite pastime as girls get a little older! Your daughter may even want to incorporate one of the following recipes into a birthday party or sleepover. Most of all, enjoy the time you spend together.

What everyone says is so true: It goes by really fast!

Here are a couple of easy recipes that you can share with your daughter:

BASIC BODY GLITTER

This is especially appealing to children around the age of six or seven.

a small, plastic container for each child, like the travel containers that you find in the drugstore or beauty-supply shop

Popsicle sticks

cosmetic-grade glitter in several colors*

vanilla extract

small paper plates

stickers

1. Give each child a Popsicle stick and a paper plate with a glob of petroleum jelly on it.

2. Have them sprinkle the glitter into the jelly and mix with the stick.

3. Add a drop of vanilla to each mixture.

4. Have each child decorate the outside of her container with stickers, then scoop the glitter into the container with the Popsicle stick.

5. Apply to cheeks, hands, etc.

*You can get sprinkle jars of micronized glitter from the art store, but cosmetic grade is ground even finer to avoid irritating the skin. It's available online at www.wholesalesup-pliesplus.com or www.handmadebeautynetwork.com.

LUSCIOUS LIP GLOSS

Fun for all ages.

petroleum jelly or beeswax (available at art-supply stores)

vanilla

lip gloss pots (either recycle yours, or purchase empty pots at a drugstore or beauty-supply store)

1. Sprinkle a few drops of vanilla into a small container of petroleum jelly.

2. Mix. (If you're using beeswax, melt it first and let it cool, then mix in the vanilla.)

3. Store the gloss in a lip-gloss pot.

Glue to the area. (Glue is commonly used in hospitals now to bind skin together.) Leave it on for a few hours until it dries thoroughly, then peel it off. It will seal the cut.

ECZEMA

Children with allergies often suffer from eczema. See page 165 for remedies.

POISON IVY OR POISON OAK

First, wash the area with soap and water, rinse, and wash it again. Some Native Americans apply a paste made from the jewelweed plant, which grows right next to poison ivy and poison oak, as cures often do. But if you don't have any jewelweed around, rub the area with the rind and flesh of a watermelon to stop the itching. You can also dab Milk of Magnesia on a cotton ball and apply to the area.

PRODUCTS: Epoch Calming Touch Soothing Skin Cream (with jewelweed) ■ Oak-n-Ivy Brand Tecnu Outdoor Skin Cleanser (wash with this immediately after contact to remove the oils that cause rash and itching).

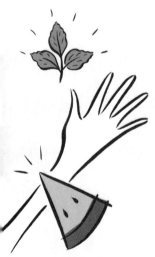

Watermelon is a great natural remedy for poison ivy.

MINOR BURNS

If a burn is severe, seek medical attention. But if the burn is minor, apply ice or a cold compress immediately. Dab lavender essential oil on the skin and keep the ice or cool compress on top until it begins to feel more comfortable. Lavender oil is amazing—it prevents blistering and calms redness, and the burn disappears without a trace.

men

In Ancient Egypt, men not only took advantage of liberal attitudes toward cosmetic use, they fought for their fair share. Workers in the Theban necropolis in the time of King Rameses III were said to have gone on strike because they didn't have enough "ointment" (what we now call a balm or moisturizer). And why not? No one should have to build a necropolis unless he can get his hands on enough hand cream to protect against dry, rough skin!

With the dawn of the "metrosexual" era, the spotlight is back on male grooming. Companies like Clinique, Jurlique, Clarins, and Neutrogena have all launched successful skincare products for men over the last few years—and guys are reaching across the medicine chest for their wives' or girlfriends' products, too. More than ever, men are realizing that good skin and a neat, well-groomed appearance is not only more attractive on a personal level, it's good for business, too. And they're going out of their way to get it.

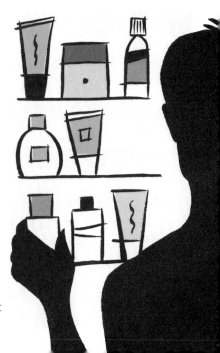

The male makeover is also happening at the spa—and the nail salon, too, where increasing numbers of men are enjoying manicures and pedicures. According to the International Spa Association (ISPA), 29 percent

SHAVE TIME

Did you know that the average man shaves off 27 feet of whiskers in his lifetime and spends a total of 3,350 hours (139 days) of his life shaving?

of all spa-goers in 2005 were male, and 63 percent of U.S. spas offer special packages for men. Men are more likely to visit a spa at their health club or on vacation at a resort spa, while women are more apt to go to the destination or day spa (where they often purchase gift certificates for men).

In any case, everybody wins: Women get the benefit of a cleaner, sweeter-smelling guy, and men get to experience the pleasures of a little pampering, on whatever level hits their comfort zone. Here are a few fast fixes to some of the most common male grooming gaffes.

RAZOR BURN

If you're prone to razor burn, don't go against the grain! Make sure your blade is clean and sharp, don't scrape too hard, and shave in the direction the hair grows, not against it. Shaving in the shower—or letting the shower run while you shave—can help soften your razor stubble and help beat the burn.

PRODUCTS: Tendskin ■ Rash Decision by Oloff Beauty.

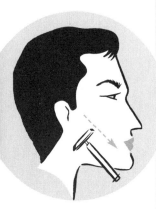

Women, don't use your guy's razor; a blunt blade can irritate his skin.

RAZOR RASH

If your skin gets sore from a blade razor, try an electric razor instead. It is gentler on the skin, since it only cuts the hair. Blade razors remove the top layer of dead skin, too, giving men a daily exfoliation.

SHAVING NICK

Rinse with cold water, and hold an alum bar or alum stick against the spot to stop the bleeding, pronto. Or, try a drop of Band-Aid Liquid Bandage to stop bleeding and create an invisible seal over the cut.

NO-DANDRUFF DANDRUFF

When some hair gels dry, they flake. Mix your gel with a dab of conditioner before you run it through your hair.

FUNKY FLAKES

Dandruff is caused by a fungus called Pityrosporum ovale, which lives on the scalp. Most of the time it doesn't cause a problem, but, occasionally, it causes dandruff. Massage cold-pressed olive oil into the scalp. Leave it on for 45 minutes, then wash the hair with a dandruff shampoo. Or, before going to bed, put some Listerine on a cotton pad, apply to the scalp, and use a dandruff shampoo in the morning.

PRODUCTS: Nizoral (inhibits growth of P. ovale fungus) or any shampoos that contain tea tree oil (available at the health-food store).

BAD BREATH

Drink a cup of black tea, which inhibits growth of the bacteria that causes halitosis, because the polyphenols in the tea destroy the bacteria. Green tea works, too, though not as well. Or, chew on a sprig of parsley or mint.

Do men need their own skincare?

Men's skin, for the most part, has different needs; it's oilier and hairier than women's, and shaving makes it tougher. So men benefit more from skincare specifically formulated for their skin. Although it's okay for men to use women's products, their fragrance, texture, and packaging may not be as appealing as products created with them in mind.

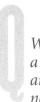

What's a scrub, and who needs it?

A scrub is a granular exfoliant that is used to slough off dead skin. Men's skin is thicker and oilier than women's, so even though men exfoliate every time they shave, using a scrub is still important, because dead skin cells can clog pores which leads to pimples and ingrown hairs. Use a couple of times a week; it leaves the face feeling smoother and paves the way for a closer shave.

WILD BROWS

Comb brows in an upward direction with a comb or a clean toothbrush, and use a small scissors to cut off any ends that are spiraling wildly out of control.

HAND HELPERS

After your home-improvement job is done, spray Pam cooking spray on your hands to remove grease or paint.

THIN, FINE HAIR

Mousse can make thin, fine hair look thicker. Apply it to palms and run them through dry hair.

THINNING HAIR

The fact is, more than 50 percent of all men will experience hair loss. If you are losing your hair, the most flattering style is to keep your hair uniformly short. In other words, nix the combover! If you choose to go the chemical route, you have three good options:

1. Propecia, a doctor-prescribed pill that will work until you stop taking it. (And don't use at all if you're trying to conceive.)

2. Topical products with minoxidil, like Rogaine. These usually work, too, until you stop.

3. Hair transplants. Consult your dermatologist or the American Academy of Dermatology for information.

INGROWN HAIRS

U se a face scrub every few days to prevent ingrown hairs from sprouting. (Tendskin will also do the trick.) If you've got an ingrown hair, put a dab of your scrub on a clean, old toothbrush, and gently go back and forth over the area. Be patient. It may take a day or two, but the ingrown hairs will lift out.

PRODUCTS: Clinique Face Scrub for Men ▪ ClarinsMen Active Face Scrub ▪ Nivea for Men Razor Defense Daily Face Scrub.

MAN WALKS INTO A SPA . . .

P hilippe Dumont started the Nickel Spa for Men, the first serious spa exclusively for men, in 1996 in Paris. In 2001, he opened a branch in New York City. According to Dumont, men are pretty clear about what they want, aside from "immediate results," of course! The top male concerns: puffiness, dark circles under the eyes, thinning hair, no shiny face, blackheads, dull skin tone, dry skin. Plus looking young, with clean and toned skin. "Men want products that give visible results along with strong sensations on the skin," Dumont says. "Of course, they don't want anyone to notice they are using skincare, so the products have to be instantly absorbed by the skin."

At the spa, the most popular treatments aren't what you might think. Men are having more facials than massage, "because they know that they need a strong cleansing," says Dumont.

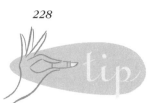

FOR MEN ONLY

When using a hairstyling product, rub it between your palms, then apply to the back of the head first, rather than the front, to prevent gooping clumping.

CALLOUSED FEET

Use a glycolic acid cream or lotion to soften the callouses. But the quickest way is to go for a pedicure—really!

DIRTY NAILS

If you work with your hands and they get dirty, soak them in warm water with lemon slices. Press your nails into the lemons, rinse, and dry.

CHAPPED HANDS

If your hands are really chapped from outdoor exposure, wet your hands and massage with oatmeal or baking soda to remove dirt, instead of using soap. Then moisturize.

COLD SORES

Apply Pepto-Bismol the moment you feel the tingle, and your cold sore will never rear its ugly head.

ROUGH HANDS

Whether you work in an office or on a construction site, chances are your hands are rough, dry, and maybe even cracked. Before you go to bed, apply hand cream. If, like many men, you hate smelly hand cream, try fragrance-free versions.

PRODUCTS: Neutrogena Norwegian Fragrance-Free Hand Cream ▪ ClarinsMen Active Hand Care ▪ Lavera Neutral Fragrance-Free Hand Cream ▪ Zim's Crack Crème ▪ Dumont Company No-Crack Hand Cream (scent-free) ▪ Porter's Lotion.

OILY, GREASY HANDS

Wash hands, then rub with cornmeal. Or, spray with a bit of Pam cooking spray, and wipe with a soft cloth or paper towels.

DRY SKIN

If your skin feels dry, ditch the soap! Wash your face with warm—not hot—water and a gentle cleanser.

PRODUCTS: Cetaphil Gentle Skin Cleanser ■ Jurlique Men's Foaming Face Cleanser ■ Decléor Jen de Billes Cleansing and Exfoliating Gel.

YOUR SKIN GETS IRRITATED SHAVING

Try shaving gel or cream, not foam, and use warm, not hot, water on your face. Let the cream sit on your face for a minute or two before shaving, and your shave will be smoother.

THE SPIKY LOOK

Hair products are essential to give a spiky style to your hair. Put some hair wax or pomade on your fingers, then comb your fingers through your hair, starting at the back of the head. You can also use a hairstyling stick—these look like stick deodorants for the hair—by running it across your fingers, then running your fingers through your hair.

PRODUCTS: Kiehl's Solid Grooming Aid ■ Bumble & Bumble Sumotech Styling Wax

GOOD GROOMING

If you have any grooming questions, log on to www.askmen.com, where you'll get a smart, well-researched response. Or try www.mug online.com, where you'll find practical, sensible advice on almost anything related to male grooming.

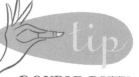

DOUBLE DUTY

Buy one clipper that will trim both nose and ear hairs!

REFRIED HAIR

If your hair feels really dry, get in the habit of using a conditioner after shampooing. Leave the conditioner on in the shower while you wash your body, then rinse. Do not use a two-in-one shampoo/conditioner; these can be drying.

BLACKHEADS ON THE NOSE

Head for the drugstore and pick up some Biore Pore Strips, or an exfoliating scrub. Or, apply a thin coat of Elmer's glue, let dry, and peel off.

ERRANT NOSE HAIRS

Take a good look in the mirror, and if you have nose hairs, buy a small nose-hair clipper at the drugstore and lose 'em—fast.

EAR HAIRS

Unless you want to look like your old Uncle Morty, clip them, wax them, or have your barber or an aesthetician at your local day spa take care of them. (Women, make it easy and get him a gift certificate.)

FUZZY WUZZY

If your hair is coarse and fuzzy, you probably wash it too much. Just because you're in the shower doesn't mean you need to shampoo. Simply rinse your hair with water or just condition it, and only shampoo every few days.

PART V:

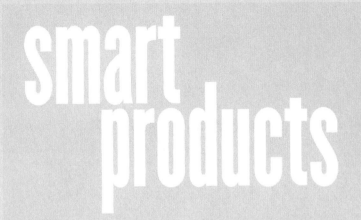

smart products

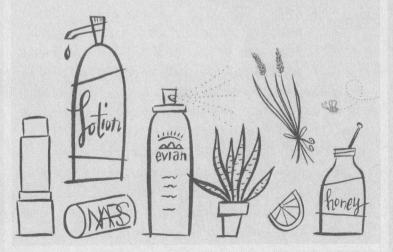

CHAPTER TWELVE

Beauty Products

A User's Guide

EAUTY PRODUCTS HOLD OUT TANTALIZING promise—and often, they deliver. What a thrill when you find a product that looks good, smells nice, and actually does what you need it to do. But with thousands launched every year, sorting the life-altering from the lame can be a dizzying experience. That's why it helps to know a few rules of the beauty game before you put yourself into play.

This chapter will tell you where to save and when to splurge on products. You'll learn about time-saving products and tools and how to use them. And you'll find out how to doctor your products—by mixing things up—to make them better suited to your individual needs.

Time-saving Products

Whether you're a working mom, a busy career woman, always in a rush, or simply a makeup minimalist, you're probably looking for ways to shave time from your beauty regimen. Here are a few easy ways to do it. (See also Chapter 2: Fast Face, pages 15–39.)

SMART PACKAGING

Certain types of packaging can save you time when you're running late for work or school in the morning. Try lotions that come out of a pump instead of a jar or tube, "pen" applicators that release concealer or nail polish with a click, hair gel that rolls onto your bangs with a mascara wand, and "roller ball" eye shadow that rolls on like a deodorant (roll it on and smudge with your fingers—no tools required).

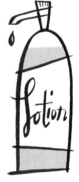

MULTITASKING PRODUCTS

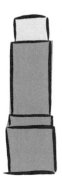

Multipurpose products are double- or triple-taskers that save time in the morning, and allow a quick transition from day into night. For example, curling mascara both curls and lengthens the lashes. Tinted moisturizer can moisturize, provide coverage, and, in most cases, offer sun protection, too. Some cream foundations dry with a silky, matte, powdery finish. Dual face and lip tints,

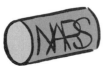

sometimes known as "multiples," will warm up both lips and cheeks, and, depending on the shade, may color your eyelids as well. These portable paints work especially well if your makeup palette is neutral. The shades are designed to enhance your natural coloring and refine a natural look. An added benefit: The packaging tends to be small, lightweight, and great on the go.

You can also gain extra mileage from other products by exercising a bit of ingenuity. In a pinch, your eye pencil can double on your brows. Or, you can dab a little lipstick on your cheeks for color.

PRODUCTS: L'Oréal Cashmere Perfect Makeup (foundation and powder in one) ▪ Benefit Cosmetics Jewels (creamy color for lips and cheeks) ▪ Lorac Portable Paints ▪ M·A·C Cream Colour Base ▪ Nars The Multiple ▪ Lola Cosmetics Sheer Lip/Cheek Pencil.

WARNING: SPOTTING RED FLAGS

Knowing your skin type will help you know what products to look for—and what to avoid. For example, if you have really sensitive skin or you're allergy prone, try to avoid products with synthetic fragrances, FD&C dyes, talc, and aluminum. If *fragrance* is in the top half of the ingredient label, that should tip you off that this product could irritate your skin. If you have oily skin, avoid potential pore-cloggers like cocoa butter, lanolin, mineral oil, sunflower oil, evening primrose oil, borage oil, shea butter, petrolatum, and coconut oil—especially if they appear in the top half of the ingredient label. And certain chemical sunscreen ingredients—like octyl methoxycinnamate and cinoxate—are often more irritating than benign blockers such as titanium dioxide or zinc oxide.

If your skin is prone to rashes and irritations, always do a patch test before you try a new product: Apply the product to a small area of your upper arm or leg, and leave on for 24 hours to make sure you don't develop a reaction.

THe Beauty DoCTor

Your new favorite product may be good, but knowing how to doctor it up (or custom-blend it for your beauty needs) can make it much better. Doctoring a product—mixing it up, toning it down, or spinning it off into another use—can make it work better, last longer, rescue it from the trash heap, and make you feel amazingly clever and resourceful. Here's how.

LIGHTEN YOUR LIPSTICK

Using your palm as a palette, take a dab of lipstick, add concealer, and mix with a lip brush before applying to your lips.

CUSTOM-BLENDED COLOR

If you have lipsticks lying around that you don't like, try mixing two together—you may create the perfect custom-blended color! Pick two discards from your makeup drawer (try to find two similar shades, i.e., two reds, pinks, or peaches). Dab a bit of each on your palm with a lip brush, mix them together with the brush, and apply to your lips. Adjust the color—or try different shades—until you've got a winner.

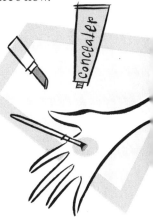

After mixing up a lighter shade, apply to lips with a lip brush.

CUSTOM-BLENDED COLOR TO GO

Store your new color (above) in a recycled eye-shadow or lip-gloss pan, or buy an empty makeup palette for your purse. Bobbi Brown's Palette can be purchased empty with room for six or eight shades.

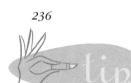

DIGITAL COLOR

Here's how to stretch your nail polish when you realize there's not enough for all ten digits. Keep a bottle of white polish on hand and mix some in with your nail-polish color. Shake the bottle well before you apply. You'll get a slightly lighter version of your original color.

CAMOUFLAGE CONCEALER

The best way to nail the perfect concealer shade is to blend it on your palm with a bit of sheer foundation.

PRODUCTS: Vincent Longo Liquid Canvas ▪ Revlon Age-Defying Light Makeup ▪ Chantecaille Future Skin Oil Free Gel Foundation.

REFOCUS

Mix two—or three—eye shadow shades together on your palm with an eye shadow brush, and apply to your eyelids.

LASTING SHINE

For fast shine, mix a silicone-based shine product with a dab of hair gel. Silicone evaporates quickly, and the gel gives it greater staying power. If your hair has a fine texture, use hair cream instead of gel.

COARSE HAIR

If your hair is dull and coarse, mix a tablespoon of baking soda and a squirt of shampoo in your palm. Shampoo, then condition. Or try an old folk remedy: Mix a capful of white vinegar in your palm with your shampoo, wash your hair, then condition.

DRAGGY CONCEALER

If your skin is dry and your concealer looks cakey, mix it in your palm with a tiny dab of foundation or a tiny bit of eye cream, then apply. It will look and feel smoother, and it will blend better into your skin.

BLUSH TOO BRIGHT

Inexpensive blush can sometimes be more heavily pigmented than more upscale, sheerer versions. If you've bought a too-bright powder blush, tone it down by blending it with translucent powder before you apply it to your cheeks.

HOMEMADE HIGHLIGHTER

To create a slightly shimmery, highlighted effect on your skin, mix a bit of shimmery gold, bronze, or pale yellow eye shadow, either cream or powder, into your foundation, then apply to your cheeks and above your brows.

LONG-LASTING LINER

Your eyeliner will last longer if you seal it with Visine. Add a few drops to a powder shadow, and stroke it on with a tiny brush, close to the lash line. (If you don't have Visine, dip a small brush into water, then into a powdered eye shadow in a matching shade, and trace over the eyeliner line.)

FOUNDATION FLAKE-OFF

If your skin is dry, it may flake around the nose after you apply foundation. To nix the flakes, mix a dab of moisturizer into a dab of foundation, and apply to the area with your fingers. (If you've got an alpha, beta, or poly hydroxy acid moisturizer handy, use it.) If you don't have moisturizer handy, gently massage lip balm into the spot.

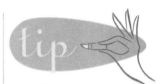

BACK BREAKOUT

If your back breaks out in the summer, be clever and use your facial sunscreen on your back. These are sheerer and less occlusive than body products, and contain fewer pore-clogging ingredients that can lend to breakouts.

DOCTOR DYE

*If your scalp stings
when you color your
hair, add two packs
of Sweet 'n Low
to the hair color
mixture before you
apply it.*

HAIR COLOR HURTS

If your scalp is sensitive, try highlighting your hair. It's less irritating to the scalp than other haircoloring techniques, because the foils create a buffer between your hair and scalp.

CHOCOLATE LOCKS

If you're a brunette and your hair color looks flat, mix a teaspoon of Hershey's unsweetened cocoa into your palm with a few squirts of your shampoo and wash your hair. It will make the color look richer, more lustrous, and, well, more chocolately! Plus, it smells yummy.

PASTY FACE

To brighten your skin, mix foundation or tinted moisturizer with a luminizer (a cream with micronized minerals, which create a bit of a gleam), or try an illuminating moisturizer.

PRODUCTS: Lorac Oil-Free Luminizer ▪ Benefit Cosmetics Hollywood Glo ▪ Prescriptives Vibrant Vitamin Infuser for Dull Stressed Skin.

TINTED MOISTURIZER A MANO

If your foundation looks and feels dry on your face, mix a dab in your palm with your moisturizer, and apply to your face with your fingers. The warmth of your body heat softens the mixture and makes it look soft and natural. (You're essentially mixing up your own tinted moisturizer.)

READ THE INGREDIENTS LABEL

Lots of chemical ingredients in beauty products exist strictly for the sake of appearances—to hold the formulation together, make it smooth, give it an appealing smell or color. But many of the peskiest skin problems—blemishes, bumps, and other irritations—can be traced back to ingredients in makeup, hair- and skincare products.

If you want to avoid problems—sensitivity reactions, clogged pores, flaky scalp—it's important to read the label on the back of your beauty products. You read food labels don't you? Even a quick glance at a cosmetic label can alert you to potentially irritating ingredients and help you assess whether you're getting a bang for your buck.

The ingredient label will tell you how much—or how little—of an ingredient is in the product, and once you know your skin type, you can spot those that you might want to avoid.

"By law, ingredients must be listed in descending order of predominance," says Rebecca James Gadberry, instructor of cosmetic sciences at UCLA Extension in Los Angeles, "from the beginning of the list down to 1 percent" (which is usually about halfway down the list). So the closer an ingredient is to the top, the more you get—and the more effective (or irritating) it will be. The controversial ingredients—preservatives, fragrances, and colors—are usually at the bottom of the list, but read carefully if your skin is sensitive or allergic.

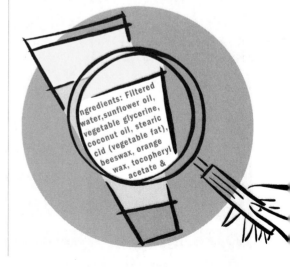

Ingredients: Filtered water, sunflower oil, vegetable glycerine, coconut oil, stearic cid (vegetable fat), beeswax, orange wax, tocopheryl acetate &

when to save,

L ike most women, you probably don't mind spending a bit more on a product, if you know that it's worth it. But the question is, how do you know? Most of us have thrown away good money on bad makeup choices. Here's a brief overview of when to save on products, when to splurge, and when to toss.

Pencils. In most cases, the biggest difference between a 99¢ pencil and a $15.99 pencil is $15. Touch the top of the pencil between your fingers; it should feel smooth, not dry. These can last a couple of years.

Blow-Dryer. With a few exceptions (the ion dryer and the Tourmaline dryer by Hairart) get an inexpensive blow-dryer. Just make sure it has a low and a cool setting. A blow-dryer will last from one to ten years.

Shampoo and Conditioner. Unless you love the smell or are hooked on "bonus" ingredients that are high up on the ingredient list, most less-expensive versions perform just as well. Hair products can last two years.

Nail Color. Unless you're drawn to an expensive shade, there's no reason to splurge on nail color. Nail polish lasts about a year or until it discolors or won't mix back together.

Sunscreen. As long as it has both UVA and UVB coverage (titanium dioxide, zinc oxide, or Parsol 1789 listed as an "active ingredient"), one sunscreen is pretty much like another. The exception is the pricey Anthelios SPF 60 which has been shown to offer amazing protection. Sunscreen loses its efficacy after a year.

Mascara. Go for an inexpensive brand like Maybelline or L'Oréal because mascara should be tossed after a few months.

when to splurge

Foundation. Foundation sits on your face all day. Many pricier brands are formulated with gentler, less-occlusive ingredients that aren't as likely to clog your pores, discolor, or fade throughout the day. Foundation can last for a year or even two.

Powder. Pricier powders last longer, which means that you get good value. Because it sits on your face for the entire day, make sure it's the best quality you can afford. Good powder lasts a couple of years.

Haircut or Color. When you're changing your style or color, splurge on a great stylist or colorist. Then, maintain the look with someone less expensive. Remember to take a photo after the initial cut to show your next stylist exactly how you want your hair to look.

Lipstick. There's no substitute for a great color—which is the best reason to splurge. Besides, cheap lipstick tends to act cheap by bleeding and feathering. When it comes to staying power, it's all about color and texture: Darker, matte shades last longest, though they tend to be most drying, while light, sheer, glossy shades are the most fleeting. Lipstick usually stays moist for up to a year.

Eye Shadow. A great color is worth more, and cheap shadow tends to be chalky. Quality shadow—which goes on smoother and lasts longer—should feel silky and creamy, not dry and crumbly. Eye shadow usually lasts up to a year.

Eye Cream. Eye cream is worth a splurge, because you want to get a formulation that's not greasy on the undereye area.

Vitamin C Cream. Vitamin C creams are hard to stabilize, cost more money to make, and therefore should cost more.

EXPIRATION DATE

Unlike food, most beauty products don't come with an expiration date. Still, there are reasonable, healthy hygiene guidelines to follow. Common sense should prevail: Toss anything that smells bad, is discolored, separates and won't go back together, or crumbles or dries out when it's supposed to be lubricious— like lipstick. Always store products in a cool place away from sunlight (not say, on the dashboard of your car) or the preservatives will break down, and it will go bad.

COLOR FORMS

If you're feeling drab, sometimes a little diversionary activity—like doctoring up your nail polish shade—can perk you up. Break up some eye shadow in your choice shade and mix it into white polish. Experiment and apply.

GO FOR THE GLEAM

Ever wonder what in the world those tubes of gold lip gloss are for? If you are a Latina or dark-skinned woman, mix a tiny dab of gold on top of your lipstick. It will warm your face and make your lips gleam.

FAST PHARMACIST

If you've got a pimple that needs immediate attention, but your nonprescription acne lotion has thickened and won't come up from the bottom of the jar, pour a few drops of alcohol-free toner in, and shake well.

FLAKY PRODUCT

You've spent good money on that hair gel and don't want to toss it, but it flakes and looks like dandruff. Mix a dab of gel with a spot of leave-in conditioner. Apply to your hair. You'll get the styling benefit without the flakes.

REACH FOR THE BRONZE

If you bought face powder that's too light, sprinkle in a bit of bronzing powder, mix and apply with a big, fluffy brush.

STRETCH your PRODUCTS

Whether you've invested time in a pampering pedicure or splurged on a pricey product, you'll want it to last. Be smart, and take advantage of these simple tricks to make your beauty products and treatments last longer. You'll save time and money.

MONTH-LONG PEDICURE

In the winter, a pedicure can last up to a month. Stretch yours by applying an extra coat of polish four days after your pedicure, and again four days after that.

TWO-WEEK MANICURE

Apply a strengthening topcoat two days after the manicure, and every other day until you get another manicure, and you can extend your manicure up to two weeks.

MOP UP THE GREASE

If you don't have time to wash your oily hair, sprinkle baby powder or dry shampoo on your brush, and brush through.

PRODUCTS: Lavett & Chin Silk & Rose Hair Powder ■ Shiseido Dry Shampoo ■ Klorane Dry Shampoo.

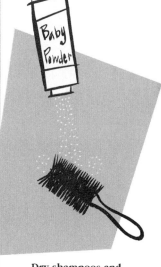

Dry shampoos and powders come in handy during extended illness or hospital stays.

DYE-LESS

If you want less-frequent hair color touch-ups, try highlights, which need to be updated only three or four times a year. Use

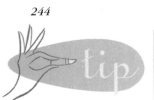

NAIL TIP

Some women have a hard time getting their polish to last. Apply vinegar to your nails before you apply your polish. It makes the polish adhere better, and your manicure will last longer.

a color-maintaining shampoo, which will extend your hair color for approximately two weeks if you're blond, three to four if you're brunette.

NO NICKS

When there's no time to shower and shave, apply body oil or massage oil to your dry legs, and shave. It moisturizes, too!

CUTICLE CRASH

When your nail polish smudges on your cuticles, and you don't have time to redo it, use these quickie products to clean it right up.

PRODUCTS: Essie Nail Corrector Pen ▪ Swabplus Cuticle Swabs Conditioner.

SMOOTH OPERATOR

If you've reached in your bag too soon and smudged your fresh manicure, try Nails AR New Dry Nail Polish Repair—it's clear, but it smooths smudgy edges and fills them in with the piled-up color nearby.

GOOD TO GLO

Before you apply your makeup, apply a moisturizing mask for five minutes. Or, massage your moisturizer into your skin for a few minutes in small, circular movements around your face.

PRODUCTS: Naturopathica Environmental Defense Mask ▪ Darphin Purifying Balm.

SHINE ON

Spray your hair with hair spray, then dip a big, pouffy powder brush into a bronzing powder or a gold or bronze eye shadow. Shake the brush to get rid of the excess and brush onto your hair, back from the hairline, to add a subtle sheen.

A Japanese-style fan brush distributes powder lightly and evenly

LIMP CURLS

To quickly rejuvenate, simply dampen your hair—using a spray bottle or your fingers—and scrunch.

SPEED DRY

Look for the Conair Ceramic Speed Styler blow-dryer, to cut back on your blow-drying time.

PRODUCT MELTDOWNS

Most of us expect a certain level of commitment from our products, just like we would with any relationship. That's why it's always a shock when they don't come through, and it's usually when you need them the most. Here's how to get what you need from your products when they're on the verge of breaking up or letting you down.

MAKEUP MELTDOWN

When your lipstick, eye shadow, and pencils soften and start to melt in

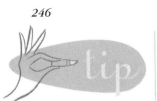

LIPSTICK FIX

To fix a broken lipstick, hold the broken sides of each half over a candle flame for just a couple of seconds (otherwise it will pick up dark soot from the candle) and press them together. Rest the lipstick on a small dish, and store it in the refrigerator until it sets.

your makeup bag, reshape them with your fingers, then store them in the refrigerator overnight.

LUMPY NAIL POLISH

Pour a drop of nail polish remover in the bottle, and shake it well.

MISSION IMPOSSIBLE

Does the cap of your nail polish bottle "glue" itself shut each time you give yourself a manicure? Waste no more time struggling with the bottle. Smudge a tiny bit of Vaseline around the top of the bottle before you twist it closed, and it will open easily next time.

ORANGE ALERT

If your makeup turns you orange, it means one of two things: (1) The color isn't right for your skin, and you need a shade with more pink in it; (2) The foundation is old and has oxidized, which causes it to discolor. Toss it.

CRUSTY MASCARA WAND

If your wand is studded with hard little bits of mascara, take a dab of Vaseline, apply to the wand with a clean finger, and wipe off the bits with a clean rag. Whatever you do, don't use soap and water to clean the wand. The soap can irritate your eyes, and the water can introduce bacteria into your mascara.

WASTED COLOR

If you lose a chunk of color whenever you sharpen your lip pencil, put the pencil in the freezer for five or ten minutes before sharpening. It will harden enough so you won't get as much color stuck in the sharpener.

THE BIG SQUEEZE

Halfway through your makeup routine, and can't squeeze another drop of tinted moisturizer or cheek gel from the tube? Grab a small pair of scissors, cut the tube open, use what you need, and scoop the excess into a travel-size mini jar for future use.

GOOD TO THE LAST DROP

If you've run out of foundation or moisturizer in the middle of putting it on, use a long-handled Q-tip (they're nice and skinny) to scrape out what you can from the bottle. Apply it directly to your face. Then, prop the bottle upside down to let the liquid slide down the sides for the next time. Better yet, buy more.

HARD AND SHINY

When oils from your face end up in your powder blush and make your pressed powder hard or shiny, scrape the surface with a small, clean kitchen knife and blow the old bits away. The makeup underneath will be soft and fresh. (A paper clip will do the trick if you're at work.)

How can I prevent my makeup from crumbling in their compacts when I carry them in my handbag?

Stash your makeup in the side zipper compartment of your bag—especially if your bag is big—or in a small makeup case. Look for products with softer packaging, for example, plastic tubes of gloss and cheek gel, and makeup packed in rubberized compacts instead of hard plastic or metal cases. Finally, the creamier a product is, the less likely it is to dry out and crack.

freebies and good stuff

T he Web is a great place to surf for beauty. And, knowing that it's difficult to read true color and smells online, many companies now offer free samples. The sites here include, "insider addresses" where you can find bargains or free stuff, philanthropic companies that combine sales with social activism, organizations that bring a bit of glamour to the needy, and just plain old good stuff at discount prices.

adiscountbeauty.com

An online beauty supply shop, with regular discounts of up to 40 percent on hair care, skincare, makeup, and more. They not only specialize in hard-to-find items, they take requests!

aedes.com

The cyber arm of Aedes de Venustas, a heavenly perfume shop in New York City. You can get seven free fragrance samples with an online purchase, or pay to sample without.

apothia.com

Even if you don't live in L.A. and get to rub elbows with celebs who shop at this trendy boutique, you can order cool beauty booty from chic retailer Fred Segal online.

beauty.com

Check out the "steals and deals" section for as much as 50 percent off perfume, skincare, bath and body products, and makeup.

beautydoor.com

You'll find boutique brands like B. Kamins Chemist, Longcils Boncza, DDF, Sothys, and Ellen Lange for up to 60 percent off.

beautyhabit.com

Check out the sample program, where you can choose six samples of different products for $1.75 each, including shipping and handling.

beauty.ivillage.com

A rotating roster of beauty samples.

beautysurvival.com

The site offers great tips for women of color, offbeat brands, and a "goodies, freebies, and specials" section that tells you where to get freebies.

blissworld.com

An online outgrowth of Bliss spas. It may take forever to get an appointment, but here's where you can get the goods. Best deal: daily bargains like a $15 eye shadow for $5.

cosmeticconnection.com

The site offers unaffiliated reviews of beauty products.

dailycandy.com

A groovy guide to stylish addresses and beauty booty in several cities.

dressforsuccess.org

An organization that offers free interview suits, makeup, and style coaching to needy women transitioning back into the workforce.

gloss.com

Anything owned by Estée Lauder—and that includes almost 50 percent

of your average department store's floor space—can be ordered here, including Clinique, Estée Lauder, Bobbi Brown, M•A•C, Prescriptives, and more.

saffronrouge.com

Devoted exclusively to organic beauty brands like Dr. Hauschka, Weleda, and more.

sephora.com

If you don't have a Sephora in your neighborhood, you can find the beauty department store online, with a wide selection of stylish boutique brands.

styleforfree.com

Everything from skincare and hair care to perfume—even toothpaste.

styleworks.org

An organization founded by Malaak Compton-Rock (Chris Rock's wife) to help women move from welfare to work. Styleworks offers free beauty services, job-interview coaching, and more. See what you can do to help.

vickerey.com

Based in Boulder, Colorado, this online shop features natural beauty products from top lines, along with workout and yoga garb, all-purpose clothing, and accessories. They feature regular sales and discounts.

CHAPTER THIRTEEN

THE NATURAL BEAUTY PANTRY

C LEOPATRA, HISTORY'S FIRST RECORDED BEAUTY queen, rubbed aloe on her face to give it a glow. In the 17th century, Mary Stuart, Queen of Scots, took advantage of the skin-softening powers of grape extract by bathing in wine. From antiquity to the present day, we've been drawn to plants and botanicals for beauty treatments.

Today, as our lives become more complicated, we're looking for simpler, more natural ways to pamper ourselves. We're drawn to the perception of purity in natural ingredients along with the belief that they are gentler and healthier for the skin. And botanicals do provide a welcome antidote to all those popular antiaging treatments, such as retinols, peels, and lasers, which can lead to irritation and sensitive-skin reactions.

For those who are interested in botanical ingredients but don't know what they are good for, here's a quick run-through of the most highly touted and most effective botanical ingredients popularized recently by the beauty industry, along with recipes for making your own products. After all, what's more natural than something that comes out of your own kitchen? However, if mashing avocado or grating ginger is not your style, but you like the idea of going natural, take advantage of the many high-quality natural products recommended in the sidebars.

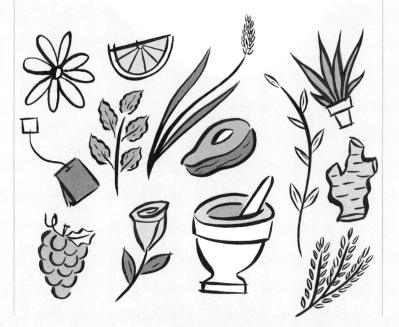

what is natural?

By law, *natural* means nothing. Although the use of the terms *natural* and *organic* have been strictly regulated by the FDA with regard to their use by the food industry, no regulations have been issued to define those terms as they apply to cosmetics.

However, a beauty product doesn't have to be 100 percent natural to contain enough of a natural ingredient to offer therapeutic benefits. But pay attention because manufacturers may hype a plant ingredient when the product doesn't contain enough to make any difference. For example, if you're buying a soothing aloe mask,

Organic?

Cruelty-free?

Natural?

Synthetic?

and aloe is listed 23rd out of 25 ingredients, chances are it's only window dressing.

Ingredients should be easier to decipher in a truly natural product. That's your first tip-off—fewer multisyllabic chemical-sounding names. Even natural products, however, need preservatives to protect them from bacteria and from oxidizing. So you're probably going to find chemical names like isopropyl-, butyl-, and propylparaben on most labels. There *are* natural preservatives—grapefruit seed extract, vitamin E (tocopherol), and vitamin C (sodium ascorbate)—but they usually only work for three to four months.

aLoe

WHaT'S IT FOr?

Aloe gel is 99.5 percent water, which is why it feels so soothing on the skin. But it also contains polysaccharides, glyco-proteins, vitamins, minerals, and enzymes that are effective moisturizers and anti-inflammatory agents. Aloe gel soothes burns (especially sunburn), moisturizes the skin, and may prevent hyperpigmentation. It also temporarily tightens the skin, which is why it's a great "mini-mask" to apply right before a big night out.

WHaT'S THe LOre?

The spiky aloe vera plant was brought from North Africa to Barbados in the 17th century, where it covered the ground in such a thicket that Spanish sailors named the islands Barbados, or "bearded." It also grows like a weed in the American Southwest.

Today many homes in Japan keep a potted aloe plant right outside the front door, and Japanese women squeeze the gel from the leaves to depuff, soothe, and cool the eyes.

ALOE PRODUCTS

■ Naturopathica Aloe Cleansing Gel

■ Derma E Aloe and Chamomile Skin Soothing Moisturizer

make your own

ALOE SKIN-FIRMING MASK
For a quick tightening mask, cut a leaf from an aloe plant. Slit it open lengthwise, and rub the exposed gel on your (clean) face. Leave on for 10 to 15 minutes, and rinse with cool water.

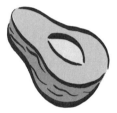

AVOCADO

WHaT'S IT FOr?

Avocado is a great moisturizer for dry skin and hair. It is rich in vitamin E and moisturizing oils, and the oil absorbs easily into the body.

WHaT'S THE LOre?

Avocado hair treatments are especially popular in Latin America, where avocado grows everywhere and is a dietary staple.

Make your own

GUACAMOLE HAIR MASK If your hair is brittle and prone to breakage, try this deep moisturizing treatment. Mash an overripe avocado until it looks ready for guacamole. Mix in an egg yolk and 2 tablespoons of olive oil. Massage it into damp hair, tuck it under a shower cap, and leave on for 15 minutes to an hour. Rinse, shampoo, and condition your hair.

CAMELLIA OIL

WHaT'S IT FOr?

Camellia oil is a common ingredient in commercial Japanese moisturizing shampoos and shine treatments for the hair. The oil is extracted from the nut of the camellia tree, a beautiful flowering plant that grows throughout Japan and is a relative of Australia's tea tree. It's a light oil that is easily absorbed into the hair shaft, and it also adds body to the hair without weighing it down.

WHaT's THE Lore?

Geishas have used camellia oil for centuries to add gloss to their long, sleek, naturally shiny hair. In Japan, women put camellia nuts in a bag and crush the nuts to release the oil. They distribute the oil by moving the bag back and forth over their hair.

CAMELLIA OIL SCALP RUB
Camellia oil is also a great moisturizer for a dry, flaky scalp. Warm ½ cup to 1 cup of camellia oil (depending on the length of your hair) in a saucepan. Dip your fingers into the warm oil, and gently massage it into your scalp with your fingertips, then rinse, shampoo, and condition. If you can't find camellia oil, use hazelnut oil instead.

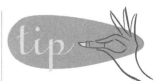

INSIDE SCOOP

Natural skincare lines like Jurlique, Osea, Dr. Hauschka Skin Care, and Naturopathica are more expensive than most, but well worth it.

CHAMOMILE

WHaT's IT For?

Chamomile is a daisy look-alike, and the flower is native to southern and western Europe. Both Roman and German chamomile (the most commonly used) contain azulene, an effective anti-inflammatory.

It soothes dry, itchy, sensitive skin; conditions the hair and brings out blond highlights; and reduces broken capillaries. A cup of chamomile tea will also soothe an achy stomach, especially after one of those triple-cappuccino mornings.

WHAT'S THE LORE?

The Victorians relied on chamomile to calm women suffering from "hysteria." Through the ages, chamomile flowers were floated in rinses used by blondes to lighten and brighten their hair after a shampoo.

BLACKHEAD-BUSTING FACIAL STEAM
To loosen blackheads, buy some loose chamomile tea in the health food store. Scatter ½ cup in a large bowl and pour boiling water on top. While it steeps, lean over the bowl, drape a towel over your head, and let your face steam. (If you're blond, reserve the liquid, pour into a spray bottle, and spray on your hair after you shampoo. It will help the sun catch your highlights.)

COCONUT

WHAT'S IT FOR?

Coconut oil absorbs easily into the hair and skin because it has a small molecular structure. It is a terrific moisturizer for the hair, but unless your skin is extremely dry, it is not recommended for skin because it can clog the pores.

WHAT'S THE LORE?

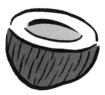

Southeast Asian women are known for their incredibly lustrous, shiny hair. The secret may be their use of coconut oil (a.k.a. monoi oil) shampoos.

Make your own

COCO LOCO CONDITIONER
Massage a quarter-size dab of coconut oil, which is available at health-food stores, into damp hair. Leave it in for ten minutes, shampoo, and condition. Your hair will be really soft and shiny.

COFFEE

WHAT'S IT FOR?

Coffee is a vasoconstrictor, which means that it can make blood vessels constrict temporarily. Its rough texture makes it effective for smoothing rough spots on the body. It is also a diuretic and is said to tighten the skin, which is why it's popular in anticellulite creams.

WHAT'S THE LORE?

Coffee is a popular exfoliant in Russia, where women bring their morning coffee grounds to the bathhouse and rub them into their skin before bathing.

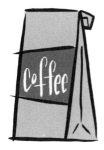

COFFEE PRODUCTS

■ Body Coffee Invigorating Body Polish

■ Jaqua Coffee Body Scrub

■ Sephora Indulgences Coffee and Cream Morning Body Scrub

JAVA JOE BODY SCRUB
In the shower, with the help of a washcloth (or your hands), massage your leftover coffee grounds all over your damp body from the neck down to slough off and soften dry, flaky skin.

EUCALYPTUS OIL
PRODUCTS

■ Essencia Eucalyptus
Therapy Aromatic
Bath Oil

■ Comfort Zone Aromasoul
Oriental Essential Oil blend

■ Bliss Hot Salt Scrub:
Rosemary and Eucalyptus

EUCALYPTUS OIL

WHAT'S IT FOR?

Eucalyptus is a common decongestant, and it's a traditional ingredient used in relaxing foot soaks throughout Asia. The eucalyptus oil helps stimulate blood flow to the area where it's applied, and it's also a topical pain reliever with analgesic properties.

WHAT'S THE LORE?

In Bali, a traditional foot bath with eucalyptus oil soothes tired feet and relieves foot pain at the end of a long day. In Asia, shoes—and, symbolically, cares and worries—are left outside the door. A foot bath then helps make the transition from a hectic to a calm environment. In Bali, fragrant tropical blooms like gardenia, hibiscus, frangipani, and ylang-ylang are floated in a eucalyptus foot soak to make it more welcoming and beautiful. After the bath, it's customary for the feet to be massaged and moisturized with coconut oil.

SKIN WARNING

If your skin is sensitive, clove, cinnamon, oregano, mint, and eucalyptus oils are apt to be irritating. If you have sensitive skin, always do a 24-hour patch test before using. (See page 234).

TIRED-TOE TINGLER

Place a layer of smooth stones at the bottom of a basin, fill it with warm water, and spike it with a few drops of clove or eucalyptus oil. Strew a few flowers in the basin, if you like. Sit and relax with your feet submerged in the water. Rotate the bottoms of your feet along the stones, grabbing them with your toes. Soak for about ten minutes. Pat your feet dry and massage with a mint- or rosemary-scented lotion, which will moisturize and re-energize your tired toes.

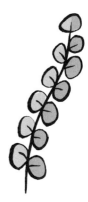

GINGER

WHAT'S IT FOR?

Ginger has been shown to be effective in treating circulatory problems because it promotes blood flow. In Thailand and other countries in Southeast Asia, pregnant women massage prai (a form of ginger) onto their bellies to prevent stretch marks. It is also a natural emollient and has been used by generations of Thai women to tone and soften the skin. Ginger is a common ingredient in body scrubs because it revs up the circulation and warms up the body.

WHAT'S THE LORE?

Ancient Romans considered ginger an aphrodisiac, and mentions of ginger spice up the stories in the classic "One Thousand and One Nights."

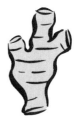

GINGER PRODUCTS

■ The Thymes Ginger Milk Body Lotion

■ Origins Ginger Body Scrub

■ Pharmacopia Ginger Body Lotion

GINGER SPICE LIP PLUMPER
To make your own lip plumper, melt 2 tablespoons grated beeswax and 1 tablespoon canola oil in a double boiler. Grate a teaspoon of fresh ginger, squeeze the juice through a piece of cheesecloth into the saucepan, and mix into the other ingredients. Store in a small lip balm tin in a cool spot.

GRAPE EXTRACT PRODUCTS

■ Caudalie Lifting Serum with Grapevine Reservatrol

■ Lancôme Vine-fit SPF 15

■ Uvavita Day Moisturizing Cream

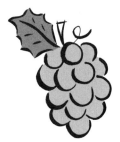

Grape extracts

WHAT'S IT FOR?

The grape—seeds, skin, and pulp—has moisturizing, antiaging properties because it is high in linoleic acid and polyphenols, a potent antioxidant. When you drink wine, you become flushed because polyphenols stimulate the circulation. Topically, grape extracts also stimulate blood flow, which feeds and nourishes the skin. The tannins in red wine are used in astringent toners and to reduce puffiness. Nothing from the grape is wasted—seeds, pulp, and skin are all tapped for use in antiaging skincare products that soften and tone skin and prevent lines and wrinkles.

WHAT'S THE LORE?

For centuries in France, wine harvesters and winemakers have been known to have the softest hands. But no one knew why until recently! At many French spas—and in

Napa and Sonoma counties, the winemaking districts of northern California—a full-body massage with fresh grapes may be found on the menu.

ANTIOXIDANT EYE CREAM
Grapeseed oil can be found in supermarkets and specialty-food shops. It's an extremely light, absorbent oil that is relatively odor free. Dab it on around the undereye area, with your fourth finger. It is a great moisturizer, and it will soften fine lines around the lips as well as remove eye makeup.

green (and white) tea

what's it for?

Green and white teas are powerful antiaging skincare ingredients and can help firm or depuff the skin. These teas are also antioxidants and anti-inflammatories, and they have been shown to inhibit pathways of inflammation in the skin. Green tea protects the skin from free-radical damage and helps make fine lines and wrinkles look smaller. It can also soothe mild eczema, sensitivity reactions, rosacea, contact dermatitis, and allergic dermatitis. Because it's such a good antioxidant, try to drink a cup of green tea a day.

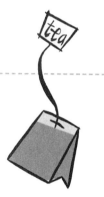

GREEN AND WHITE TEA PRODUCTS

- Origins A Perfect World For Eyes
- EO White Tea and Rose Moisturizer
- Replenix CF Cream

WHAT'S THE LORE?

Chinese poets in the fifth century called green tea "froth of the liquid jade" and gave it a place of honor in the Zen tea ceremony. Japanese women brew green tea tonics to lift, firm, and soothe the skin.

Make your own

GREEN TEA DEPUFFER
To depuff the undereye area, prepare 2 cups of green tea (use tea bags). Let them steep for about five minutes. As the tea cools, remove the tea bags and chill them in the refrigerator. When cool, give them a gentle squeeze, lie down, and apply to the undereye area for about ten minutes. Pour the tea in an ice cube tray, freeze, and apply to eye area when tired or stressed.

HONEY PRODUCTS

■ Red Flower Japanese Peony Moisturizing Body

■ Gardener's Greenhouse Clover Honey Hand and Body Lotion

■ Burt's Bees Milk & Honey Body Lotion

HONEY

WHAT'S IT FOR?

Honey isn't, technically, a botanical, but it's such a common ingredient in natural care that I had to include it. Honey helps the skin retain moisture, which is why it's such an effective ingredient for dry skin. It is also an anti-inflammatory and soothes irritated skin.

WHAT'S THE LORE?

Honey is often used as a moisturizer by inhabitants of mountain villages in northern India and Pakistan, where temperatures drop quite low in the winter, and dry skin is a problem.

 HONEY FACE MASK Warm 1 cup of honey in a saucepan. Cleanse and exfoliate your face, then brush a thin layer of warm (not hot!) honey onto your face with a small brush or your fingers. Leave on for ten minutes. Rinse gently with warm water and a washcloth. Your skin will feel sweet!

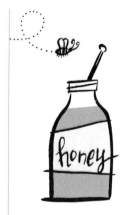

JEWELWEED

WHAT'S IT FOR?

Jewelweed calms red, itchy, or irritated skin.

WHAT'S THE LORE?

Native Americans believe the cure can often be found growing next to the scourge, which is true in the case of jewelweed. It grows next to poison ivy in dry, arid places, where it is used by certain tribes as an antidote to poison ivy.

 SOOTHING POULTICE If you can find fresh jewelweed, pulverize the leaves with a mortar and pestle, and apply directly to itchy, irritated skin.

JEWELWEED PRODUCTS

■ Epoch Calming Touch Soothing Skin Cream

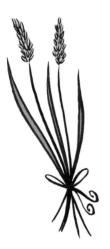

LAVENDER

WHAT'S IT FOR?

In 1920, Dr. Rene-Maurice Gattefosse, a French chemist, discovered that lavender not only had antimicrobial and anti-inflammatory properties and healed burns, but the scent had a calming effect on the nervous system. Lavender also kills the bacteria that cause acne, and it's great in a relaxing evening bath because it calms the nerves and helps you sleep.

WHAT'S THE LORE?

The word *lavender* comes from the Latin *lavare* ("to wash"), which is appropriate since the Ancient Romans used it in the bath to relax and soothe tired muscles. In the Elizabethan era—when housekeeping and personal hygiene left a lot to be desired— lavender buds were strewn on the floor so that they would release their scent and perfume the air when walked upon.

LAVENDER PRODUCTS

- Kneipp Lavender Bath Salts Thermal Skin

- Pharmacopia Lavender Bath Salts

- Weleda Lavender Body Oil

Make your own

LAVENDER BATH SALTS Pour a cup of coarse-grained or kosher salt into a bowl. Add 1 cup of Epsom salts, and 1 cup of baking soda. Add up to 15 drops of lavender essential oil (depending on how strong you like the scent) and ¼ cup of sweet almond oil. Mix thoroughly, store in a glass mason jar, and scoop into a warm bath (with a small seashell, if you like) as needed.

LEMON

WHAT'S IT FOR?

Lemon is an excellent exfoliant for flaky skin on elbows and knees. The scent of lemon provides an invigorating wake-up call, and it's an energizing ingredient in bath oils and bath gels. Because lemon juice reacts so strongly to sunlight, it's also a great highlighter for the hair during the summer.

WHAT'S THE LORE?

"Citrus limon" was known as "the golden apple" in the days of Alexander the Great, and it was passed as a gift among kings. Ancient Egyptians used lemons to treat food poisoning. In Ancient Rome, where blond hair was always desirable, women streaked their hair with lemon juice. In the court of Louis XIV, women used lemons to redden their lips and splashed on lemon eau de toilette for its refreshing scent.

Make your own

MOP-UP MASK To make a mask that will cleanse and tone oily skin, slice a lemon in half. Scoop out enough pulp from one half to fit an egg yolk inside. Place the egg yolk in the lemon cup and refrigerate overnight. Apply the lemon-infused egg yolk to clean, dry skin, avoiding the eye area. Leave on for ten to 15 minutes. Rinse with warm water.

SKIN WARNING

Citrus oils (grapefruit, lime, lemon, orange, bergamot, and neroli) can be photosensitive, so don't go out in the sun right after using them.

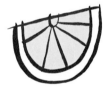

LEMON PRODUCTS

- Bliss Lemon Peel

- Jaqua Girls Sinfully Rich Lemon Meringue Body Butter

- Avalon Organic Botanicals Lemon Hand & Body Lotion

- Fresh Sugar Lemon Body Lotion

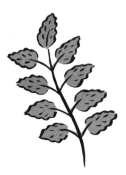

MINT PRODUCTS

- Naturopathica Peppermint
  Tea Tree Foot Balm

- The Body Shop Peppermint
  Foot Lotion

- Lotil Peppermint
  Foot Cream

- Florestas Foot Cream
  (with rosemary, peppermint,
  tea tree, and plant butters)

MINT

WHAT'S IT FOR?

Peppermint and spearmint are both commonly used to rejuvenate tired, achy feet. Mint reduces inflammation and relaxes muscles. It feels cooling and smells refreshing— a great pick-me-up for those down dogs. Mint contains menthol, which cools the skin, increases the blood flow, and is an antibacterial.

WHAT'S THE LORE?

Mint was brought to the U.S. from England, where it thrives in moist spots, like river banks. In Ancient Greece and Rome, it was used medicinally to warm and stimulate the circulation, and to soothe nauseous, upset stomachs.

FRISKY FOOT BATH Fill a basin with cool mint tea, toss in a couple of ice cubes (and a sprig of mint as a pretty accent) and soak for a few minutes.

NEEM OIL PRODUCTS

- Dr. Hauschka Skin Care
  Neem Nail Oil Pen

- Sundari Neem
  Essential Oil

NEEM OIL

WHAT'S IT FOR?

Neem oil is an antifungal and antibacterial oil that comes from a tree indigenous to

India. It is a terrific moisturizing treatment for dry nails and cuticles, but be forewarned, Neem does have a strong smell.

WHaT'S THE Lore?

Neem is a staple ingredient used in Indian ayurvedic beauty treatments for dry hands and feet, and as a treatment for athlete's foot.

Make your own

CUTICLE CREAM Buy a small tin of shea butter and mix in a few drops of neem oil. Massage into dry, cracked cuticles.

nuT BuTTers anD OILS

WHaT'S IT FOr?

Nut butters are nonirritating, rich, occlusive moisturizers that are especially soothing to irritated or sensitive skin. In Brazil, the home of the microthong and the bikini wax, indigenous nut and butter oils are used as overall body moisturizers, and to soothe skin after waxing. These occlusive butters restore the barrier function of the skin that's stripped away during waxing. Sweet almond oil works as an extremely absorbent moisturizer on its own, or as the base for many gentle skincare products.

NUT BUTTER AND OIL PRODUCTS

- The Body Shop Body Butter

- Weleda Almond Intensive Facial Cream

- Alba Hawaiian Body Polish Sugar Cane

- Florestas Buriti Fruit Lotion Botanical

- Florestas Cupuacu Seed Butter Hair Conditioner

WHaT'S THe Lore?

The Amazon rain forest in Brazil is the source of many vitamin-rich nuts that not only sustain the diets of indigenous people but keep Brazilians looking good, too. Cupuacu butter, brazil nut oil, and babassu oil act as anti-inflammatories and soothe irritated skin.

Make your own

BUTTER SKIN SOOTHER
Warm a bit of nut butter or oil in your palm and let your body heat soften it. Gently massage into affected areas.

OLIVE OIL PRODUCTS

- Baronessa Cali Oliva Tarocco Firming Face Cream
- Mediterranean Spa Olive Oil Body Butter

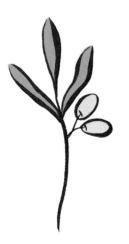

OLIVE OIL

WHaT'S IT FOr?

Olive oil is an excellent moisturizer that's also light and gentle enough for sensitive skin. A beauty staple for centuries in Mediterranean climates, it is used to moisturize the skin and hair and as a base oil in body scrub treatments at spas around the world.

WHaT'S THe Lore?

Olive oil, extracted from the fruit of the olive tree, is known as "liquid gold" in Italy, because its health and beauty benefits are priceless. Italians mix it with blood orange or lemon juice to create moisturizing treatments for the skin and hair.

THREE-IN-ONE FACIAL Do what Italian women do for a one-step cleansing, exfoliating, toning, and moisturizing treatment that brings a healthy glow to the skin. Mix ¼ cup of olive oil in a bowl with the juice or finely grated skin of an orange or lemon (citric acid causes surface cells to slough off). Massage the mixture gently into the face and rinse with cool water.

PAPAYA

WHAT'S IT FOR?

Papaya fruit is indigenous to tropical climates around the world, where it is pulverized and used in face masks, to nourish and moisturize the skin. The enzyme papain exfoliates rough, dull-looking, dead skin, and evens out skin tone. It also contains antioxidant vitamins A and C, which repair damaged skin and fight free radicals. It's good for aging or oily skin, or for those with adult acne.

ANTIAGING MASK Take a quarter of a papaya, cut it in pieces, and put in the blender with ¼ cup of yogurt. Gently massage into cleansed face, and leave on for ten minutes. Rinse with warm water.

PAPAYA PRODUCTS

- Paw Paw Ointment

- Derma E Papaya Soy Foaming Facial Cleanser

- Astara Green Papaya Nutrient Mask

RICE PRODUCTS

- Fresh Rice Face Cream
- Rice blotting papers
- Komenuka Bijin Moisture Cream

RICE

WHAT'S IT FOR?

The rice milk mask is a colloid, a pasty material like oatmeal that has a drying effect like a poultice, helping to cool the skin and draw out oil.

WHAT'S THE LORE?

In China, pulverized rice is a common ingredient in face powders and blotting papers, which absorb oil and reduce shine. "Rice milk—the starch that comes up from the rice after it's left in water—is used to help soak up oil from the face," says Jamie Ahn, of the Acqua Beauty Bar in Manhattan.

Make your own

JAMIE AHN RICE MASK Let rice soak in warm water for 30 minutes. Pour off the water and mix it with soy flour or rice flour until it forms a paste. Apply to clean, dry skin, leave on for ten minutes, then rinse with cool water.

FOLLOW YOUR NOSE

Much of the benefit of botanical ingredients comes from inhaling their lovely aromas. But smells mean different things to different people. Learn to make substitutions: If eucalyptus, rosemary, or sage are suggested to stimulate your slothlike body but you don't like their scents, use peppermint or spearmint as a substitute.

ROSE

ROSE PRODUCTS

- Neal's Yard Remedies Rose & Almond Night Cream

- Dr. Hauschka Skin Care Rose Day Cream

- Chantecaille Flower Harmonizing Cream

WHAT'S IT FOR?

Rose oil is a great moisturizer for dry, mature, sensitive, or aging skin. Rose oil constricts small blood vessels and reduces redness and broken capillaries. Rose water—with no alcohol added—is a gentle, natural astringent. In aromatherapy circles, the smell of rose oil is said to ease anxiety, make you feel good, and promote feelings of love.

WHAT'S THE LORE?

In ancient times, a rose hanging over a meeting table meant that the meeting would be held in strict confidence, or sub rosa. Rubbing a woman's hips with rose oil was supposed to ease the pain of childbirth in the Middle Ages, perhaps by lessening the laboring woman's anxiety. Cleopatra seduced Marc Antony by carpeting her floors in rose petals, and Nero favored rose-petal baths.

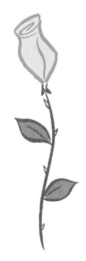

Make your own

ROSE WATER TONER Simple rose water—available at many grocery and specialty-food stores—makes a great toner. Keep it chilled, sprinkle it on cotton or gauze, and use it to blot excess oil from your face. Or pour it into a mini spray bottle and spritz your face. It's particularly gentle and soothing on sensitive skin.

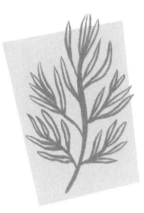

ROSEMARY PRODUCTS

- Aura Rosemary Mint Shampoo

- Weleda Rosemary Hair Oil

- Avalon Organic Botanicals Volumizing Rosemary Shampoo

ROSEMARY

WHaT'S IT FOr?

Rosemary adds shine to the hair, espe-cially if you're a brunette. It stimulates the scalp and hair follicles, and controls flak-iness and dandruff.

WHaT'S THe LOre?

Rosemary is a bushy evergreen with spiky leaves. It is related to mint, sage, basil, and patchouli. The leaves have a strong scent and were used as incense by the Ancient Egyptians.

ROSEMARY HAIR TONIC
Boil 2 cups of water. Pour the water over 1 cup of chopped fresh rosemary leaves. Let steep until cool. Rinse your hair with the mixture after shampooing.

SAGE PRODUCTS

- Lavett & Chin Clary Sage, Rose & Neem Shampoo

- Dr. Hauschka Skin Care Sage Bath

- Weleda Sage Deodorant

SAGE

WHaT'S IT FOr?

Sage oil kills bacteria and microbes, which is why, before refrigeration, it was used to protect meat from spoiling. It is antiseptic and astringent, controls excess oil secretion, regenerates skin cells, and kills bacteria that cause body odor and acne.

WHAT'S THE LORE?

Sage is considered an important herb by Native Americans, who burn it in purification ceremonies and sweat lodges and use it to cleanse a room. Its detoxifying properties are thought to heal disease by driving out evil spirits, because disease was often seen as a spiritual affliction. Sage proliferates in the American Southwest and around the Mediterranean.

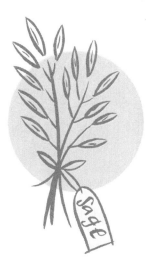

SAGE BACNE BUSTER A sage bath is a good way to treat body acne, because it balances excess oil. A sage-and-oatmeal soak will also soothe irritated skin. Fill a muslin bag or a square of cheesecloth with ½ cup of oatmeal and 2 tablespoons of fresh or dried sage leaves. Tie it closed with string or a ribbon and hang it under the faucet while water is running. Soak in the bath, then remove the bag and gently press against your back.

SEAWEED (AND ALGAE)

WHAT'S IT FOR?

Seaweed is rich in vitamins (A, C, and K), minerals, and fatty acids, which moisturize and remineralize the skin. It has antioxidant properties, too, which protect the skin from free radical damage.

SEAWEED AND ALGAE PRODUCTS

- Osea Atmosphere Protection Cream

- Charles Tipton Seaweed Mask

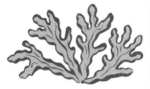

WHaT'S THE Lore?

The therapeutic properties of the sea are legend, especially in coastal areas of Europe, where inhabitants went to "take the cure" from the ocean's healing waters and bracing salt air. They also went to the sea to treat respiratory and skin conditions.

Make your own

SEAWEED SOAK Buy a package of nori (the seaweed used to roll sushi) at the supermarket. Cut three sheets into squares, place them in a small pot, and fill with water. Let it boil for five minutes, cool, and pour into your bath.

SESAME OIL PRODUCTS

■ Neutrogena Sesame Body Oil

■ Avalon Organic Botanicals Moisturizing Body Oil

SESAME OIL

WHaT'S IT For?

Because its molecular structure is small, sesame oil is considered one of the most deeply penetrating oils. It's rich in linoleic acid and fatty acids, which carry water-soluble nutrients through the skin. Use it as a moisturizer for dry skin and hair and as a rub for dry and cracked nails.

WHaT'S THE Lore?

Sesame oil has been used in Indian ayurvedic medicine for 5,000 years. Sesame oil is a food oil—pressed from the seeds of an Asian plant— and, according to ayurvedic beliefs, you should be able to eat anything you apply to your body.

 SESAME BODY SCRUB To make a moisturizing body scrub, toast 1 cup of sesame seeds in the toaster oven to release the oil and make your scrub more fragrant. With a mortar and pestle, crush seeds with 1 cup of sea or kosher salt. Add ½ cup of sweet almond oil and mix. Massage into damp skin and then shower.

SHEA BUTTER

WHAT'S IT FOR?

Shea butter is rich in vitamins A, E, and F, which protect the skin from free radicals, help prevent lines and wrinkles, and moisturize dry, heat-damaged, overprocessed hair. It's a luxurious moisturizer and a great humectant, which draws moisture into the hair and coats the shaft to make hair soft and supple.

WHAT'S THE LORE?

Shea butter comes from the nut of the karite tree, which grows wild on the west coast of Africa. In Ghana, women use shea butter to take down ashiness in the skin and soothe their aching feet. It's also used as a cooking oil before it hardens into the butter that's applied to skin and hair.

SHEA BUTTER PRODUCTS

- L'Occitane Shea Butter Hand Cream
- Carol's Daughter Tui Shea Butter Hair Smoothie
- Frédéric Fekkai Shea Butter Hair Mask
- Philip B African Shea Butter Shampoo

HAIR SILKENER Look for "whipped" shea butter, which is formulated so that it's light and easy to apply. Before your shower, scoop out a handful from the jar and massage it through dry hair. Leave on for up to 30 minutes. Rinse, shampoo, and condition your hair.

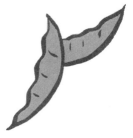

SOY

WHAT'S IT FOR?

Soy is used to soften brittle, damaged hair and moisturize aging skin. It can also make the skin look brighter and even out mottled skin tone. Shampoos and conditioners with soy coat the hair follicle and make it more flexible and better able to retain moisture.

WHAT'S THE LORE?

Throughout Asia, soy, a rich, nourishing protein and a dietary staple is commonly found in beauty products.

SOY TIGHTENING MASK Mix ½ cup of finely ground soy flour with an egg white. Apply it to a cleansed face, and leave on for ten minutes. Rinse with cool water. Moisturize.

TEA TREE OIL

WHaT'S IT FOr?

In Australia, tea tree oil is a renowned blemish-buster. The pungent, astringent oil is commonly dabbed on blemishes with a Q-tip or cotton pad. It's an anti-inflammatory, an antibacterial, and an antiseptic. Its acidic quality enables it to exfoliate and unclog pores. Tea tree oil is also used to treat dandruff and soothe itchy insect bites. Despite all its therapeutic uses, some people find the smell of tea tree oil offensive. So take a whiff before purchasing.

WARNING: Do not use it if your skin is sensitive or allergic.

WHaT'S THe LOre?

Tea tree oil is extracted from the leaves of the tea tree, which grows in swampy coastal regions of Australia. Aborigines crush the leaves and apply a poultice directly to wounds and skin infections.

Make your own

ACNE TREATMENT It's easy to find tea tree oil at health-food stores. Use a Q-tip and apply the oil directly to blemishes. Since its smell is so strong, mix a few drops of lavender essential oil into the tea tree oil to tone it down before you dab it on blemishes. Always avoid the eye area.

TEA TREE OIL PRODUCTS

- Ole Henriksen Roll-On Blemish Attack
- Burt's Bees Herbal Blemish Stick
- Desert Essence Natural Facial Cleansing Pads
- Samuel Parr Aromatherapy Correcteur Pen

Index

m

n

Q, r